A WOMAN'S GUIDE
TO VITAMINS, HERBS,
AND SUPPLEMENTS

OTHER ST. MARTIN'S PAPERBACKS TITLES
BY DEBORAH MITCHELL

The Complete Book of Nutritional Healing

*Consumer's Guide to Prescription and Over-the-Counter
Weight-Loss Supplements*

The Diet Pill Guide

The Dictionary of Natural Healing

Nature's Painkillers

The Broccoli Sprouts Breakthrough

A WOMAN'S GUIDE
to Vitamins, Herbs, and Supplements

DEBORAH MITCHELL

Foreword by Hunter Yost, M.D.

A Lynn Sonberg Book

St. Martin's Paperbacks

NOTE: If you purchased this book without a cover you should be aware that this book is stolen property. It was reported as "unsold and destroyed" to the publisher, and neither the author nor the publisher has received any payment for this "stripped book."

Notice: This book is intended as a reference volume only, not as a medical manual. The information given here is designed to help you make informed decisions about your health. It is not intended as a substitute for any treatment that may have been prescribed by your doctor. If you suspect that you have a medical problem, we urge you to seek competent medical help.

Mention of specific companies, organizations, or authorities in this book does not imply endorsement by the author or publisher, nor does mention of specific companies, organizations, or authorities imply that they endorse this book, its author, or the publisher.

Internet addresses given in this book were accurate at the time it went to press.

A WOMAN'S GUIDE TO VITAMINS, HERBS, AND SUPPLEMENTS

Copyright © 2008 by Lynn Sonberg Book Associates.

Cover photo © Steven Poe/Workbook Stock.

All rights reserved.

For information address St. Martin's Press, 175 Fifth Avenue, New York, NY 10010.

ISBN: 0-312-94510-8
EAN: 978-0-312-94510-7

Printed in the United States of America

St. Martin's Paperbacks edition / January 2009

St. Martin's Paperbacks are published by St. Martin's Press, 175 Fifth Avenue, New York, NY 10010.

10 9 8 7 6 5 4 3 2 1

CONTENTS

PART II: SUPPLEMENTS

VITAMINS AND MINERALS

AMINO ACIDS AND MISCELLANEOUS SUPPLEMENTS

PART III: YOUR PERSONAL SUPPLEMENT PLAN

FOREWORD

The health concerns of women are unique and require unique attention from their doctors. Women in general are more proactive about their health than men, and it is ironic and sad that health issues affecting women such as heart disease have been underappreciated by the medical profession for many years. Virtually all of the major diseases affecting women, such as breast cancer, lung cancer, heart disease and osteoporosis, are preventable with dietary and lifestyle changes. Specific nutrients such as vitamin D are extremely important in preventing these same diseases. Dietary changes emphasizing plant-based proteins rather than animal proteins can be helpful for menopausal symptoms and heart disease. Certain herbs and B vitamins can be important for balancing and metabolizing hormones. A variety of minerals are important for bone health, in addition to calcium. Other herbs can help reduce pain and inflammation. A hormone from the adrenal glands, DHEA, converts to both estrogen and testosterone and can improve energy, moods and libido in middle-aged women. It can also be used by itself as a form of hormone replacement for some women but should be measured in the blood by your doctor. Some women should not take it if they are prediabetic.

The information in *A Woman's Guide to Vitamins, Herbs, and Supplements* can give women options concerning the now-controversial hormone replacement therapy. Women can and should be as informed as possible about their health.

Try to find a doctor who is knowledgeable in nutrition or at least open-minded to your concerns and ideas. This timely and practical book can help women take immediate charge of their health.

Hunter Yost, M.D.
www.hunteryostmd.com

INTRODUCTION

In this book, we have gathered the latest information on nutritional and herbal supplements that can effectively tackle the health challenges faced by women today. At this moment, which health issue personally concerns you the most? Is it heart disease? As the number one killer of women in the United States, with one-third of all women dying of the disease, it certainly warrants your concern. How about breast cancer? It affects one in eight women and is the second most common cancer among women. Are you haunted by PMS? Up to 90 percent of women experience some degree of premenstrual syndrome during their lifetime. These and many other health concerns can have a dramatic impact on your everyday life and the lives of those closest to you.

Although it's true that the majority of health issues discussed in this book can affect men (with obvious exceptions), they all have features that are unique or special to women only. Did you know, for example, that the warning signs and symptoms of a heart attack are different for women than they are for men, or that the cause of a headache or migraine for women is typically different than it is for men? Similarly, some natural supplements are especially for women only. For example, you won't see a man taking black cohosh capsules or sipping red clover tea. In many cases, the needs of men and women for the same essential nutrients also differ greatly. A good example is folic acid: Although both men and women need this nutrient, it is especially critical for women of childbearing age to help prevent birth defects, and women who are pregnant or breast-feeding need higher amounts.

The Natural Supplement Revolution

Since you picked up this book, we're betting you're part of the natural supplement revolution. Or perhaps you're getting ready to join. In either case, you are not alone.

Americans spend more than $19 billion a year on natural supplements, an amount that has increased steadily since the early 1990s and continues to do so today. One reason these alternative products remain so popular is that more and more people are dissatisfied with over-the-counter and prescription medications and the side effects they cause, which can often be more debilitating than the conditions being treated. Another reason is that many conventional medications fail to provide relief from ailments, diseases, and symptoms ranging from sniffles and cough to menstrual cramps, arthritis, migraine, varicose veins, memory problems, and heart disease. Many women, for example, are turning to herbal remedies to fight the symptoms of PMS and menopause, enjoying the benefits of products with names such as red clover, chaste tree berry, and chamomile. These and other plant remedies have a long history of relieving such symptoms among women in many cultures.

People turn to natural supplements because it makes them feel like they have some control over their health. Indeed, the fact that you picked up this book indicates that you want to take charge as well. Taking control, however, requires that you do some homework and talk to qualified health care professionals, as needed, who are well versed in the unique health needs of women so they can help you decide which natural supplements can meet your health and wellness goals. This book is one important tool you can use to assist you as you make those decisions.

Why You Need Nutritional Supplements

According to the Centers for Disease Control and Prevention, four of the top six leading causes of death in the United States are related to diet. This is both a disheartening statement and a promising one. It's disheartening because although we have access to many delicious and nutritious foods, many people have such a fast-paced lifestyle they do not take the time to eat them.

Yet even if you are conscientious about eating nutritious food, you may find it difficult to meet your goals every single day. Unexpected guests, having to work late, illness, travel, car trouble, family demands—so many things can try to get in the way. That's one reason why taking nutritional supplements, starting with a basic multivitamin/mineral, is so important. Here are a few more reasons:

- Many foods are grown in nutritionally depleted soils, which means the harvested plants do not contain the levels of nutrients they should. Buying only organic produce is one way to avoid this problem, but it is not always available and it can be too costly for some people.

- The American diet consists primarily of processed, refined foods that have been depleted of many of their nutrients.

- Processed foods contain chemical additives that place stress on the body and impair its ability to absorb nutrients.

- High levels of emotional and/or physical stress promote imbalance in the body and the development of nutritional deficiencies and disease.

If you are like most women, you take or plan to take nutritional supplements because you want to improve or maintain your overall health and/or prevent illness, especially if you are pregnant or planning to have a child, and there are many studies that support these reasons. Researchers have evidence, for example, that multivitamins can lower the risk of cardiovascular disease and diabetes, help prevent weight gain, and reduce the risk of certain cancers, including colon cancer. A University of North Carolina at Chapel Hill study is just one of several that found lower rates of preterm births among women who took multivitamins prior to conception and during pregnancy. Some experts have documented lower rates of infection among elderly people who take multivitamin/mineral supplements. The list goes on and on.

Many people also turn to individual nutritional and herbal supplements to treat specific symptoms or medical conditions, and with good reason: A growing amount of research shows us that taking such supplements along with a healthy diet and lifestyle can help prevent scores of health problems, fight disease, and improve physical and mental health. In the United States, some of the most popular supplements are black cohosh, calcium, garlic, ginkgo, ginseng, green tea, glucosamine, omega-3 fatty acids, St. John's wort, and vitamin C. People buy these and other natural products to treat menopause, PMS, headache/migraine, colds and flu, arthritis, depression, and heart disease, among other health problems. And they, like you, are turning to books such as this one to help them decide which supplements may work for them.

Natural Does Not Equal Safe

When you hear the phrase "natural supplement" or "herbal supplement" do you automatically think "Oh, I know they're safe"? If so, you're not alone. Many people equate the words "natural" and "herbal" with "risk-free," believing that a vitamin or herbal remedy couldn't possibly harm them, no matter how much they take. The truth is, anything you take in excess—even water—can be detrimental to your health. If you misuse herbs or nutritional products, side effects may occur. At the same time, nutritional and herbal supplements can have a very significant, positive impact on your health, which is why we encourage you to take such products in the amounts recommended by knowledgeable health care practitioners, reliable literature, or product labels.

How to Use This Book

So, are you ready to take charge of your health using natural supplements? Do you want to know more about your health challenges and how you can better prevent, treat, and manage them naturally? Then read on to find out how this book can help you.

In Part I, we invite you to explore nearly fifty medical and health conditions that concern women today. Chances are you picked up this book because you are looking for natural alternatives to conventional medicine to prevent or manage health or medical conditions that are affecting your life or perhaps the lives of other women that are close to you. We chose the conditions in this section based on the impact they have on women's lives and whether natural supplements could reasonably be expected to help prevent and/or treat them. In each entry you will find background information on the condition, causes and risk factors, and a list of "Best Bets" and "Other Options," which are the natural supplements that have been shown to help prevent, manage, and/or treat the ailment. Although we provide suggested dosages for each supplement, you are then encouraged to turn to the corresponding entries in Part II, where we offer detailed information on each of the supplements.

We round out each entry in Part I with a section called "Of Special Interest to Women," where you can learn how women experience a disease or condition differently than men or discover special or unique characteristics about the condition that may help you better manage it. Suggested readings and references that support the information in the entry can be found in the "For Further Reading" section at the end of the book.

In Part II, you can learn which natural supplements (vitamins and minerals, herbal remedies, and amino acids and miscellaneous nutrients) you can incorporate into your lifestyle to support and promote health and well-being and to prevent, manage, and/or treat medical conditions that affect your life. In each entry, you will learn basic information about the nutrient, how to take it as a supplement, food sources, and specifically its benefits, including the medical and health conditions discussed in Part I. Again, each entry also includes the segments "Of Special Interest to Women," and more information can be found in the "For Further Reading" section.

In Part III, we invite you to use the knowledge you've gathered from parts I and II to build a personal supplement program. Don't worry, we help you create it in three easy steps: (1) choose a multivitamin/mineral, (2) customize your plan by adding supplements that address your specific needs (we provide an extensive checklist to help you), and (3) learn how to decipher supplement labels and how to buy and use herbs. We round out the chapter with a few recipes that feature some of the natural supplements discussed in the book.

Overall, this book serves as a comprehensive, convenient guide to the natural supplements that can help you and all women take more control of your health and well-being.

PART I
Women's Medical and Health Concerns

ACNE

Approximately 75 percent of adolescent girls and at least 12 percent of women have to face it: the pimples, bumps, cysts, redness, and inflammation that greet them in the mirror not just for a day or two but for weeks, months, even years. Acne, also known as acne vulgaris, is a chronic skin condition that affects approximately 60 million Americans, according to the American Dermatological Association. Acne is not just a teenage phenomenon: 20 percent of adults have active acne, and up to half have at least one episode during adulthood.

Although acne can range from mild to severe, it all begins the same way: oil glands (sebaceous glands) in the skin secrete an oily substance (sebum) into the hair follicles. The sebum lubricates the hair and skin, but if too much sebum is produced, it can block the skin pores and trap dead skin cells. A plug then forms and develops into a closed comedone (whitehead) or open comedone (blackhead). If bacteria get into the comedones, the skin becomes inflamed and pimples form. Sometimes pimples fill with pus (in which case they're called pustules) and invade deep into the skin, forming painful sacs called cysts. Because pustules and cysts form scar tissue when they heal, they can leave pits in the skin.

Causes/Risk Factors

Acne typically first appears during adolescence and is largely caused by hormonal changes. These changes stimulate the sebaceous glands to increase sebum production, a process that usually subsides by age 20. Yet acne can also appear for the first time in adults, and here the cause may be a genetic predisposition, hormonal changes (especially related to menstruation or high testosterone levels), use of certain prescription medications (e.g., lithium, corticosteroids, oral contraceptives, phenytoin), or a reaction to certain cosmetics.

Prevention and Treatment

Although there are no known ways to prevent acne, you can significantly reduce its severity and impact if you:

• Use mild soap when you wash your face.

• Avoid use of cosmetics that contain oil, which can clog your pores, or those that contain lanolin, isopropyl myristate, sodium lauryl sulfate, laureth-4, D&C red dyes.

• Wash your hair frequently.

• Avoid irritating or picking any pimples.

• Eat a whole-foods diet that includes four to five servings of green vegetables daily (chlorophyll is good for the skin) and lots of fiber.

Perhaps you've heard the expression "feed your skin," and that's what natural supplements can do. Be patient, however, as it can take 6 to 8 weeks before you see significant results.

Best Bets

- *Vitamin A or beta-carotene.* Up to 25,000 IU (see the box on page 244 for unit conversion) daily of vitamin A is considered safe for postmenopausal women; a comparable dose of beta-carotene is 30,000 mcg. For women who are pregnant or who could become pregnant, take no more than 10,000 IU daily of vitamin A or 6,000 mcg of beta-carotene.

- *Tea tree oil.* When applied to acne, it may reduce bacteria and improve symptoms, including inflammation. Compared with benzoyl peroxide, tea tree oil gel is just as effective but has fewer side effects (e.g., burning, dryness, stinging, itching). Apply a drop or two to each lesion three times daily or use 5% gel twice daily.

- *Vitamin B complex.* Two to three times daily, take 25 to 50 mg. Also include extra vitamin B_6—take 25 mg twice daily for severe acne, once daily for mild to moderate acne. One study also found that women with premenstrual acne alleviated acne flare-ups before their menstrual cycles when they took 50 mg of vitamin B_6 daily.

Other Options

- *Copper and zinc.* Begin with 30 mg zinc twice daily for three months, then reduce zinc to once daily and add 1 mg copper daily, because long-term zinc use can reduce copper levels.

- *Aloe vera.* Squeeze the gel from the leaves of this plant or use a commercial gel that contains aloe vera to soothe your skin. Apply as needed.

Of Special Interest to Women

Blame it on hormones: Adolescent girls and women of all ages are much more likely than men to experience mild to moderate acne, according to a 2008 study in the *Journal of the American Academy of Dermatology*. For some women, hormone fluctuations two to seven days before the menstrual period begins can trigger an outbreak of acne. Women who have polycystic ovary syndrome typically also have high levels of testosterone, which may cause acne. Other hormonal changes that can trigger acne include pregnancy, starting or stopping birth control pills, or hormone therapy. Recent research also indicates a relationship between DHEA levels and acne in women (see "DHEA").

If you are pregnant and have acne, be especially careful, as many of the medications used to treat acne, including retinoids, isotretinoin, and the antibiotics tetracycline, minocycline, and doxycycline, can harm the fetus.

ADRENAL FATIGUE
Adrenal fatigue is a syndrome—a collection of signs and symptoms—that develops when the adrenal glands become overburdened and no longer can efficiently produce hormones. Typically adrenal fatigue occurs in three stages: (1) the adrenal glands respond to stress by increasing the secretion of adrenal hormones, including adrenaline and cortisol; (2) when stress is chronic or persistent, it causes excessive production of certain hormones, especially cortisol, in an attempt to alleviate the damage to the body caused by the stress; (3) when the adrenal glands can't make enough cortisol in response to chronic stress, they become fatigued and cortisol levels drop excessively low. Throughout this process many symptoms can occur, ranging from mild to debilitating.

Cortisol's most important function is to help the body respond to stress, be it physical (e.g., surgery, infections), emotional, and/or environmental, by converting proteins into energy, fighting inflammation, and releasing glycogen for energy. It also helps the body recover from infection, maintain blood pressure, and regulate metabolism of fats, proteins, and carbohydrates. When cortisol performs these duties for a short time, as it was designed to do, the body usually responds well. If, however, chronic stress keeps cortisol levels high, then cortisol attacks the body and weakens the immune system. The result is adrenal fatigue.

Many physicians do not recognize adrenal fatigue and so it is often undiagnosed or misdiagnosed. An expert on adrenal fatigue, Dr. James Wilson, author of *Adrenal Fatigue: The 21st Century Syndrome,* notes that approximately 80 percent of people in North America experience adrenal fatigue at least once during their lifetime. For some people it is a temporary condition, lasting only a few days or weeks; for others, it lingers for months or years.

One way to help diagnose adrenal fatigue is the ACTH (adrenocorticotropic hormone) challenge test. When this hormone, which is made by the pituitary gland, is injected into the body, an increase in adrenal hormone should occur. If it does not, adrenal fatigue is a probable diagnosis.

Causes/Risk Factors

Adrenal fatigue can be caused by genetics or by various stressors, including nutritional deficiencies, chronic physical and/or emotional stress, exposure to environmental toxins (e.g., secondhand smoke, household solvents, pesticides, food preservatives), use of stimulants (e.g., caffeine, nicotine, alcohol, sugar, cocaine), and chronic infections, especially respiratory (e.g., bronchitis, pneumonia).

Regardless of the cause, adrenal fatigue can leave you with tiredness, muscle weakness, swollen fingers and/or toes, swollen lymph nodes in the neck, intolerance to cold, low blood pressure, joint and muscle pain, constipation, sleep disturbances, depression, and allergies, among other symptoms. Fortunately, adrenal fatigue can be prevented and treated successfully using a natural approach.

Prevention and Treatment

Your best defense against adrenal fatigue is a nutritious diet, adequate sleep, conscientious stress reduction and management, and avoidance of toxins. Temporary adrenal fatigue, which is caused by stressors, will respond to lifestyle changes and supplementation. Permanent cases, which can result from surgical removal of the pituitary or adrenal glands, congenital adrenal hyperplasia, or Addison's disease, require hormone replacement but can also benefit from nutritional supplements. A stress reduction program is strongly recommended to go along with any supplement program.

Best Bets

- *Vitamin C.* Taking 3,000 mg daily can help reduce elevated cortisol levels, psychological stress, and blood pressure, according to several studies.

- *DHEA.* When the adrenal glands are overworked, they lose their ability to produce adequate DHEA. Supplementation with DHEA may also help protect against overproduction of cortisol by the adrenal glands. Have your DHEA levels checked before beginning supplementation (see "Of Special Interest to Women"). A typical dose is 20 to 50 mg per day.

- *Vitamin B$_5$ (pantothenic acid).* Vitamin B$_5$ plays a key role in adrenal health and is necessary for the production of cortisol. The recommended dose is 1,500 mg daily.

- *Magnesium.* This mineral plays a major role in adrenal function. Supplement with magnesium aspartate, 100 to 300 mg daily.

Other Options

- *L-theanine.* This amino acid increases the body's levels of gamma-aminobutyric acid (GABA), a neurotransmitter that promotes relaxation and a sense of well-being, and also helps to restore sleep. A suggested dose is 100 to 400 mg daily.

- *Asian ginseng.* Ginseng can improve adrenal function, reduce high cortisol levels, and improve the ratio of cortisol to DHEA to a healthier balance (see "DHEA"). A suggested dose is 100 mg twice daily.

- *Melatonin.* A nightly dose of 2 mg of melatonin can help balance the DHEA/cortisol ratio, which is important for adrenal health. This hormone can also regulate sleep and reduce stress.

Of Special Interest to Women

Adrenal fatigue affects both men and women, although it is more common among middle-aged women. This trend may be related to hormone fluctuations that occur as women move into menopause.

One of the hormones that declines with age is DHEA, which is a precursor to critical hormones, including progesterone, estrogen, and testosterone. DHEA supplementation is often recommended for adrenal fatigue, but you should consult your doctor and have your DHEA levels checked before taking the hormone. DHEA levels should be monitored during treatment to make sure the hormone is being metabolized properly. Improper DHEA supplementation can cause male characteristics, including deepening of the voice, facial hair, and hair loss. It may also cause acne, insomnia, headache, weight gain, and abnormal menstrual cycles.

AMENORRHEA

The absence of menstruation—whether during puberty or later in life—is called amenorrhea. Females who have not started menstruating by age 16 have primary amenorrhea; those who were menstruating but stop having periods for three months or longer have secondary amenorrhea. Secondary amenorrhea is much more common than the primary form, and usually the cause is not serious. Pregnancy, for example, is a cause of secondary amenorrhea.

Amenorrhea is also a sign of other conditions and situations (see "Causes/Risk Factors"). In addition, depending on the cause of amenorrhea, women may experience headache, vision changes, excessive hair growth on the face and/or torso, and a milky discharge from the nipples.

Causes/Risk Factors

In many cases, the cause of primary amenorrhea is unknown. Possible reasons include dysfunction of the ovaries, abnormal formation of the reproductive organs, and problems with the pituitary gland and/or the brain and central nervous system. Secondary amenorrhea may be attributed to use of contraceptives, breast-feeding, stress, medication (e.g., antidepressants, antipsychotics, some chemotherapy drugs), chronic illness, hormonal imbalance, polycystic ovary syndrome, low body weight, excessive exercise, thyroid dysfunction (hypothyroidism), pituitary tumor, scars on the uterus (due to Caesarean section or uterine fibroids), and premature menopause.

Prevention and Treatment

If you experience amenorrhea, consult your gynecologist to determine the cause, even if you think you know the reason. She or he may recommend you undergo a hormone evaluation and/or complete physical examination.

Because amenorrhea is a sign and not a disease in itself, treatment involves addressing the underlying cause, such as hypothyroidism or hormone imbalance. Stress reduction and improved nutrition can go a long way toward correcting amenorrhea, as can natural supplements.

Best Bets

- *Calcium, magnesium, and vitamin D.* Regardless of the cause of amenorrhea, protect yourself against bone loss by taking these bone-sustaining supplements: calcium, 1,000 mg daily in divided doses; magnesium, 500 mg in divided doses and two hours after calcium; and vitamin D, 400 IU daily.

- *Chaste tree berry.* This herb balances prolactin (high prolactin levels are a sign of amenorrhea), helps regulate the menstrual cycle, and increases progesterone production. An effective dose is 40 drops of extract in water, taken daily for six months.

Other Options

- *Vitamin B_6.* May reduce high prolactin levels. Dose is 200 mg daily.

Of Special Interest to Women

It is tempting to view the premature cessation of your menstrual period as a benefit (goodbye cramps, pads, and tampons), but there's a downside: Bone density loss and the increased risk of osteoporosis could be a major concern if you experience amenorrhea for more than three or four months. Therefore, make sure you get adequate calcium, magnesium, and vitamin D and talk to your doctor about how to maintain your bone health.

ANEMIA

Anemia is a general term for a condition in which there is insufficient oxygen in the blood. The most common form of anemia—and the one that affects women most often—is iron-deficiency anemia, which we focus on here.

Iron-deficiency anemia occurs when there isn't enough iron in the blood to manufacture hemoglobin, the substance in red blood cells that transports oxygen from the lungs to the rest of the body. Twenty percent of women of childbearing age have this type of anemia. Iron-deficiency anemia can be difficult to detect during the beginning stages because the symptoms mimic other conditions. Some of those symptoms include headache, loss of appetite, pale skin, shortness of breath during exercise, fainting, weakness, sore tongue or mouth, brittle nails, rapid heartbeat, and fatigue.

Causes/Risk Factors

The main cause of anemia in women is menstrual bleeding. Normally, women of childbearing age lose 20 to 40 mg of iron every month during menstruation. This fact, combined with an insufficient intake of iron from food and/or supplements, can result in iron-deficiency anemia. Other causes include gastrointestinal bleeding, pregnancy, parasites, recurring infections, and poor absorption of iron due to digestive disorders, poor diet, use of diuretics, or kidney problems. One risk factor for iron-deficiency anemia you can control is diet: A diet that contains few iron-rich foods or foods that interfere with iron absorption can put you at significant risk for anemia.

Prevention and Treatment

You can help prevent iron-deficiency anemia if you watch your dietary iron intake. Foods with the highest iron values include liver and other organ meats (go organic if you choose these foods), but other sources include beans (e.g., black, kidney, lima, chickpeas, lentils), brown rice, clams, dried fruits (e.g., prunes, raisins, apricots), enriched cereals, nuts, oysters, and pumpkin seeds. Foods that interfere with iron absorption should be eaten in limited quantities, including uncooked kale and spinach, almonds, coffee, black tea, and colas. Eating the following foods with iron-rich foods will enhance iron absorption: broccoli, brussels sprouts, cantaloupe, green and red bell peppers, oranges, orange juice, tomatoes, and white wine.

Smart diet choices, along with iron and other complementary supplements, can very effectively treat iron-deficiency anemia.

Best Bets

- *Iron.* The iron supplement that is best absorbed and most gentle on the gut is ferrous peptonate, followed by ferrous chelate and gluconate. Always take iron supplements with food. Have your iron levels checked before beginning supplementation. A typical dose is 100 mg daily, but allow your physician to determine the best dose for your needs.

- *Vitamin C.* Take vitamin C along with your iron supplement to enhance absorption of iron. Dose: 500 mg daily.

Other Options

- *Dandelion.* This herb may enhance your body's ability to absorb iron from food and supplements. Try 5 to 10 mL of tincture in water three times daily.

- *Vitamin A/beta-carotene.* Include vitamin A or beta-carotene to help you digest the iron in your supplement. Dose: 5,000 IU daily.

Of Special Interest to Women

Some women develop iron-deficiency anemia because of heavy bleeding from fibroids or unopposed estrogen syndrome. If you experience heavy menstrual flow, consult your gynecologist to determine the reason.

If you have anemia and are pregnant, you are not alone: Anemia affects more than 50 percent of pregnant women. This is not surprising once you know that pregnant women require 50 percent more iron than nonpregnant women (the DRI for pregnant women is 27 mg; for nonpregnant women ages 19–50, 18 mg; for women 50+, 8 mg). Iron deficiency anemia is also more common among women who have already given birth, especially if the children are close in age.

A cautionary note about choosing iron-rich foods is in order. If you are pregnant, avoid eating liver, as it can contain up to ten times the recommended amount of vitamin A, which can be toxic to a developing fetus.

ANOREXIA NERVOSA

Anorexia nervosa is a serious, often life-threatening psychological disorder that can take a tremendous toll on the entire body. This eating disorder is characterized by a distorted body image, rejection of food, and an obsession with being thin, coupled with an extreme fear of getting fat. More than 90 percent of the people with anorexia are female, and the disease typically affects adolescent girls and women in their early 20s and may go on for years, even decades, if not treated. Anorexia nervosa is defined as a loss of 15 percent or more of body weight, which individuals achieve through various means, including refusing to eat, excessive exercise, self-induced vomiting, and/or abuse of diuretics, laxatives, and enemas.

With the dramatic loss of weight often comes a litany of symptoms of malnutrition, including bloating, constipation, dry skin, dehydration, muscle cramps, thinning hair, irregular heartbeat, depression, anxiety, downy hair on the face and other areas, and cessation of the menstrual cycle. For 5 to 20 percent of women with anorexia, the organ damage caused by the disease is fatal.

Causes/Risk Factors

Experts agree that there is no one cause of anorexia, and that the reasons why people develop anorexia are largely associated with societal expectations and psychological factors rather than physical ones, although genes and hormonal changes may have a role. Research shows, however, that a major cause of anorexia is intense pressure for women to be thin. A history of sexual abuse or rape, a mother or sister with anorexia, a strong desire to be perfect, or a difficult mother-daughter relationship also may be contributing factors.

Prevention and Treatment

There are no clear ways to prevent anorexia. If you have a family member or someone else close to you who has signs or symptoms of anorexia, you may try to gently but firmly express your concern and offer to help. People who are anorexic typically strongly resist advice and deny anything is wrong, so patience and persistence are in order.

Treatment typically includes both nutritional and psychiatric therapy, such as cognitive behavioral therapy, family therapy, and nutritional counseling. Depending on the severity of the condition, people with anorexia may be treated as an inpatient at a facility or as an outpatient. Anorexics are usually in a state of starvation (a catabolic state), and the body compensates by decreasing its need for many nutrients. This reduced need for nutrients helps preserve the body and so nutrient deficiencies are usually not seen in anorexics. However, damage continues in all the organ systems. Once nutritional treatment begins, including an increase in caloric intake, the following supplements may be helpful.

Best Bets

- *Zinc.* Add some zing with zinc, which can enhance recovery from anorexia. A five-year study of zinc in anorexia found that zinc supplements resulted in weight gain, improved mental state, and better body function, plus an 85 percent remission rate. A 2006 report from the University of British Columbia recommends that all people with anorexia take 14 mg of zinc daily for two months.

- *Calcium and magnesium.* To help restore and maintain bone density, take calcium and magnesium. Magnesium is also critical for heart health, which is compromised in many women who have anorexia. Anorexics who use diuretics are often magnesium-deficient, as these drugs deplete the mineral from the body. Dose: 1,500 mg of calcium (calcium carbonate or phosphate) taken in two divided doses with meals. For magnesium (magnesium lactate or chloride), take 750 mg in two divided doses between meals.

- *Vitamin C.* This vitamin boosts the bioavailability of magnesium. Take 500 to 1,000 mg daily in divided doses along with magnesium.

Other Options

- *DHEA.* Women with anorexia tend to have low levels of DHEA, which is important for bone mineral density. DHEA should be used only under a physician's supervision. A typical dose is 5 mg three times daily, with gradual increases up to 50 mg daily if needed.

- *Dandelion.* This herb can stimulate appetite. Dose: 5 mL of tincture in water two to three times daily.

Of Special Interest to Women

Women can be especially hard hit by anorexia. Cessation of menstruation (see "Amenorrhea"), for example, is common and can result in a serious loss of bone density and a high risk of osteoporosis and bone fracture. A lack of menstruation also can cause infertility.

Women who are anorexic and who use laxatives, diuretics, or weight loss drugs during pregnancy can harm the developing child, as these substances deprive the child of necessary nutrients and fluids. Pregnant women who are anorexic also are at risk for premature labor, miscarriage, labor complications, and diabetes, as well as for low-birth-weight infants or infants who suffer from delayed growth.

Up to 40 percent of anorexic women also develop bulimia, in which they repeatedly go on eating binges and then rid themselves of the food through self-induced vomiting and/or the abuse of laxatives, diuretics, or other substances.

ANXIETY DISORDERS

A small amount of anxiety can be positive: It can sharpen your ability to cope with or manage stressful situations. But when anxiety becomes obsessive or overwhelming, when it is accompanied by a sense of impending doom or intense fear and disrupts your daily activities, then it is a disorder. Unfortunately, anxiety disorders are not rare; in fact, they are the most common mental illness in the United States. According to the Anxiety Disorders Association of America, an estimated 40 million Americans suffer from an anxiety disorder, yet only one-third get treatment.

Anxiety disorders can be broken down into six categories:

- *Generalized anxiety disorder.* People experience unrealistic, excessive worry that lasts six months or longer. Accompanying symptoms may include trembling, insomnia, abdominal pain, dizziness, irritability, and muscle aches.

• *Panic disorder.* This disorder is characterized by severe attacks of panic that can make you feel as if you are having a heart attack or are going crazy. Other symptoms may include heart palpitations, chest pain, a choking feeling, fear of dying, fear of losing control, feelings of unreality, sweating, and trembling.

• *Social anxiety disorder.* People with this disorder have extreme anxiety about being judged by others or doing something that is extremely embarrassing. Physical symptoms may include heart palpitations, blushing, profuse sweating, and faintness.

• *Post-traumatic stress disorder (PTSD).* This disorder can develop after someone has experienced a traumatic event, such as rape, witnessing a death, a natural disaster, or going to war. People with PTSD may "relive" their traumatic event through nightmares or flashbacks, avoid places that remind them of the trauma, or shut down emotionally and withdraw from others. Other symptoms of PTSD may include insomnia, poor concentration, and irritability.

• *Obsessive-compulsive disorder.* Individuals who have this disorder suffer with persistent, recurring thoughts (obsessions) that reflect excessive anxiety or fears—for example, an unrealistic fear about being contaminated by everything in the environment. Such people may then perform rituals or routines (compulsions), such as washing their hands repeatedly, to rid themselves of the contamination and thus their anxiety.

- *Phobias.* A phobia is a persistent, irrational fear of an object, situation, or image that has a negative impact on quality of life and can even be incapacitating.

Causes/Risk Factors

Anxiety disorders can be caused by a variety of factors, and often more than one applies. Stress from life circumstances (e.g., death of a spouse or friend, loss of a job, divorce, changing jobs, financial crisis, major surgery, loss of living quarters) is a major anxiety producer. An imbalance of hormones and/or brain chemicals, including serotonin, estrogen, or progesterone, can cause anxiety. Nutritional deficiencies, food or chemical sensitivities or allergies, and excessive use of caffeinated beverages or foods can also be factors.

Risk factors for anxiety disorders include being female (see "Of Special Interest to Women"), extreme shyness during childhood, family history of anxiety disorders, untreated depression, poverty, cultural pressures, and lack of social support, among others.

Prevention and Treatment

One of the most effective anxiety reducers is exercise. Regular participation in activities you find enjoyable, perhaps walking, aerobics, yoga, or qigong, can significantly reduce anxiety and thus prevent advancement to anxiety disorder. Other ways to prevent anxiety include following a nutritious diet, getting adequate sleep, and practicing stress reduction.

Supplements can be used either alone or to complement your efforts plus any conventional medical treatment, which typically includes antipsychotic and/or antidepressant drugs.

Best Bets

- *St. John's wort.* Take for anxiety associated with depression. A typical dose is 300 mg two to three times daily.

- *Black cohosh.* For anxiety especially associated with menstruation. Dose: 40 to 80 mg daily in tablets or a liquid extract (40 drops). If you prefer a tincture, the dose is 0.4 to 2 mL of a 60% ethanol tincture daily.

- *Inositol.* Panic attacks and obsessive-compulsive disorder may be alleviated by taking inositol. A starting dose is 500 mg twice daily, with increases up to 12 g per day as needed.

Other Options

- *Magnesium.* A natural stress reducer. Dose: 250 to 600 mg daily, in divided doses.

- *Calcium.* Complement the magnesium with 600 to 1,200 mg daily, in divided doses. Take the supplements two hours apart.

- *Vitamin C.* To alleviate a panic attack, take vitamin C, which reduces elevated cortisol levels associated with such attacks. Suck on vitamin C lozenges for quick results.

Of Special Interest to Women

Women are twice as likely to be afflicted with general anxiety disorder, panic disorder, and phobias, and also are affected by PTSD more than are men. Although obsessive-compulsive disorder is seen equally among women and men, one group especially at higher risk is women who have just given birth.

Postmenopausal women are more likely to have a panic attack than their younger counterparts, while pregnancy appears to have an impact on panic disorder, improving it for some women while making it worse for others. Anxiety during pregnancy may be associated with elevated estrogen levels, which may be alleviated with milk thistle and vitamin B complex: two capsules of milk thistle with breakfast, along with 25 mg of B complex, is suggested. At the same time, avoid caffeine and refined sugar.

ASTHMA

More than 30 million Americans have asthma, a chronic respiratory disease that involves recurring attacks of breathlessness usually accompanied by wheezing, tightness in the chest, and coughing. Such episodes may be triggered by any number of things, ranging from foods to environmental factors or emotional issues.

During normal breathing, the airways to the lungs are open. If you have asthma, however, a trigger causes the lining of the airways to become clogged with mucus and to become inflamed as the muscles around the airways tighten.

Causes/Risk Factors

Experts don't know exactly what causes asthma, but there appears to be a hereditary component. You may be born with asthma but not know it until you are exposed to elements that trigger your symptoms. Such triggers may include air pollutants (e.g., pollen, mold, secondhand smoke), cold weather, or fumes from perfumes or chemicals. Certain medications, including aspirin and other anti-inflammatory drugs as well as beta-blockers, can worsen asthma attacks.

Risk factors for asthma include being female (more women than men have the disease); having allergies, including allergies to airborne substances and/or foods;

exposure to pollution, including secondhand smoke; a family history of asthma; and certain medical conditions, including gastroesophageal reflux and respiratory infections.

Prevention and Treatment

If you have asthma, avoiding known triggers is the best way to prevent attacks. For the majority of people with asthma, those triggers are airborne. Therefore, installing HEPA filters in your home, vacuuming often, having everyone remove their shoes when entering the house, and having your ducts and vents cleaned professionally at least once a year can help you breathe easier.

Treatment of asthma with natural supplements can be quite effective. Here are a few recommendations.

Best Bets

- *Omega-3 fatty acids.* These essential fats can reduce inflammation and have improved asthma symptoms in adults. A suggested dose is 1,000 mg daily.

- *Quercetin.* This flavonoid can inhibit the production and release of inflammatory and allergic substances, such as histamines. Quercetin supplements are available with bromelain, another anti-inflammatory agent, and help with absorption. Try taking 1,000 to 2,000 mg daily in three divided doses.

- *Vitamin C.* This vitamin can reduce the severity of attacks. A suggested dose is 500 to 1,000 mg one to three times daily, depending on your tolerance. Take your last dose before retiring to alleviate early morning asthma attacks.

Other Options

- *Lycopene.* Limited research has shown that this phytonutrient can provide relief from exercise-induced asthma. A suggested dose is 30 mg daily.

- *Butterbur.* This herb contains petasins, chemicals that inhibit histamines. Studies show that asthmatics who used butterbur had fewer and less severe asthma attacks, and 40 percent of patients needed less medication while taking butterbur. A typical dose is 50 to 150 mg daily.

- *Boswellia.* This herb may reduce the number of attacks. In a double-blind, placebo-controlled study, participants took 300 mg of boswellia three times daily for six weeks; 70 percent improved, compared with only 27 percent of patients who took a placebo.

Of Special Interest to Women

Asthma affects women differently than men. Some adolescent girls experience a worsening of asthma symptoms when they first go through puberty. These symptoms usually return to normal once menstrual cycles have stabilized. In young women, asthma significantly increases the risk of developing obstructive sleep apnea, which causes poor sleep and daytime drowsiness.

If you are pregnant and have asthma, it is critical that you control your symptoms. Any reduction in the oxygen level in your blood can cause your fetus to get less oxygen as well, which may impair your child's development.

Two other factors to consider if you have asthma are menopause and osteoporosis. Changing hormone levels at menopause may cause asthma symptoms to worsen. These changes typically improve over time. Having asthma also increases your risk of developing osteoporosis. This increased risk is associated with the use of steroids or high doses of inhalers over a prolonged time.

BACK PAIN

Seventy to 85 percent of Americans experience back pain at some time during their life, according to the National Institutes of Health. The lower back is by far the most common area affected, and the pain can range from mild to severe, annoying to disabling, dull to sharp, and intermittent to persistent. Lower back pain often restricts movement and interferes with normal activities.

Signs and symptoms of lower back pain include pain, tenderness, and stiffness in the lower back; pain that radiates into the legs or buttocks; discomfort or pain while sitting; weakness or fatigue in the legs while walking or standing; and difficulty standing erect or standing in one position for a long time.

Causes/Risk Factors

Most back pain is caused by long-term neglect: years of poor posture, lifting incorrectly, lack of exercise to strengthen back and stomach muscles, obesity, and unmanaged stress. The results of such neglect can be a pulled muscle, an inflamed tendon or ligament, a ruptured disc, or an irritated sciatic nerve, all of which can result in back pain.

Risk factors for back pain include obesity, poor posture, work that requires a significant amount of bending and lifting, lack of exercise, smoking, pregnancy, arthritis, depression, and anxiety.

Prevention and Treatment

The number one way to help prevent back pain is to strengthen your back and abdominal muscles, as they help stabilize your back. Exercises to strengthen these muscles can be found in books and on videos and can be learned from a physical therapist or other health professional. Other preventive measures include the following:

• Learn to lift and carry objects properly; see the Mayo Clinic's, "Protect Your Back While Lifting," http://www.mayoclinic.com/health/back-pain/LB00004_D&slide=1.

• If you sit for extended periods of time, get up about once every hour and stretch your back.

• Practice good posture. Don't slouch, make sure your desk is at the proper height, and sleep on your side with knees bent.

• If you are overweight, lose weight.

• Incorporate stretching and back-strengthening exercises into your lifestyle.

Exercise is one of the best treatments for back pain, but before you start an exercise program, talk to your doctor to make sure you don't do anything that could harm your back. Natural supplements can complement your efforts.

Best Bets

• *Magnesium.* People with chronic low back pain have responded well to magnesium, as it may relieve muscle spasm and regulate muscle contraction. A typical dose is 700 to 1,000 mg daily, balanced with 1,500 to 2,000 mg of calcium. Take the two supplements two hours apart.

• *Bromelain.* This potent anti-inflammatory may offer relief with a suggested beginning dose of 2 to 3 grams daily (on an empty stomach), then reduced to 1 to 2 grams as pain diminishes.

• *Capsaicin cream.* When applied to the skin, capsaicin depletes substance P, a neurochemical that transmits pain. A normal dose is 0.025 percent capsaicin cream used four times daily.

Other Options

• *MSM.* For chronic lower back pain and muscle spasms, MSM has been effective in some patients. A suggested starting dose is 4 g (1 level teaspoon of powder dissolved in water) daily, with increases up to 20 g daily as needed.

• *Vitamin D.* Researchers at the University of Minnesota found that 93 percent of 150 people with chronic musculoskeletal pain had a vitamin D deficiency. Taking 5,000 to 10,000 IU of vitamin D daily for three months may significantly reduce back pain.

• *Vitamin B$_{12}$.* A double-blind Italian study found that vitamin B$_{12}$ can significantly reduce back pain and the need for medication. An effective dose is 800 to 1,000 mcg daily, sublingual tablet.

Of Special Interest to Women

Women are more prone to certain types of back pain. For example, women who have fibromyalgia and/or osteoporosis frequently experience back pain. Tailbone pain, or coccydynia, afflicts more women than men, and part of the reason is that it is associated with pregnancy, which places increased pressure on the lower spine.

Speaking of pregnancy, back pain during pregnancy is common, yet if it lasts for several weeks or months, this is an indication that it may persist postpartum, and you should take steps to treat it immediately. Talk to your doctor about an exercise and treatment program that can alleviate the pain during pregnancy and prevent it from becoming a chronic problem.

BREAST CANCER

Breast cancer is a malignant tumor that originates in the breast cells. It is the second most common form of cancer in women (nonmelanoma skin cancer is number one). The U.S. Cancer Statistics Working Group reports that in 2004, more than 186,000 women were diagnosed with breast cancer and nearly 41,000 lost their battle with it. Overall, one in every eight women is affected by the disease.

Not all breast cancer is the same: It can be invasive or noninvasive, and there are variations of each type, although some are rare. It is possible to have a combination of cancer types. Brief descriptions of the four most common types are below.

- Invasive ductal carcinoma (IDC) is the most common type of breast cancer, accounting for 80 percent of invasive breast cancers. IDC begins in a duct and then invades the fatty tissue of the breast, after which it may spread to other parts of the body (metastasize).

- Invasive lobular carcinoma (ILC) starts in the lobules (milk-producing glands) and can spread to other parts of the body. About 10 percent of invasive breast cancers are ILCs.

- Ductal carcinoma in situ (DCIS) is a noninvasive breast cancer and the most common of this type. It represents about 20 percent of all new breast cancer cases and is characterized by cancer cells inside the ducts that have not spread into surrounding tissue.

• Lobular carcinoma in situ (LCIS) begins in the lobules and stays within their walls. Women who have this type of cancer have a higher risk of developing an invasive breast cancer.

Causes/Risk Factors

Risk factors for breast cancer fall into two categories: things you can change and things you can't. Risk factors you can change include being overweight, using birth control pills, drinking alcohol, not having children, having your first child after age 35, using hormone replacement therapy, smoking, and eating a high-fat diet. Risk factors you cannot change include your age (the chance of getting breast cancer increases as you get older), beginning your period before age 12, going through menopause after age 55, having certain genes that greatly increase risk (BRCA1, BRCA2), and having dense breasts.

Although experts have identified many risk factors for breast cancer, they do not yet fully understand how they prompt cells to become cancerous. So far, changes in DNA appear to play a role in these changes, but much more research is needed.

Prevention and Treatment

You can reduce your risk of developing breast cancer by acting on the risk factors you can change; that is, maintain a healthy body weight, get regular exercise, avoid alcohol, don't smoke, and avoid using hormone therapy. You can also practice early detection—breast self-exams, mammograms, professional breast exams—which give you a chance to catch the disease early enough to increase your chances of successful treatment.

Some natural supplements may help prevent breast cancer or complement conventional treatment by improving quality of life and relieving side effects.

Best Bets

• *Flaxseed.* Some studies suggest the lignan in flaxseed may bind to estrogen receptors and thus help reduce the risk of breast cancer. The usual dose is 30 to 50 g daily of flaxseed.

• *Green tea extract.* This contains epigallocatechin-3-gallate (EGCG), which studies show can inhibit the activity of breast cancer cells. Researchers also found that women with early-stage breast cancer who drank at least five cups of green tea daily before their diagnosis were less likely to have a recurrence of the disease after they completed treatment. As a supplement, the recommended dosage is 300 to 400 mg of standardized green tea extract daily.

• *Melatonin.* Studies suggest this hormone may inhibit the growth of certain types of breast cancer cells, and it may enhance the effects of some chemotherapy drugs, including tamoxifen. If you have breast cancer, consult with your doctor before starting melatonin.

Other Options

• *Folic acid.* A dose of 400 mcg daily is recommended, especially for women who drink alcohol. One study of more than 50,000 women found that adequate intake of folic acid may reduce the risk of breast cancer associated with alcohol use. Another found that women who had a high folic acid intake (an average of 456 mcg daily) had a 44 percent lower risk of invasive breast cancer than women who had a low intake (160 mcg).

- *B complex.* A high-potency supplement is recommended because B vitamins activate folic acid plus help control stress.

Of Special Interest to Women

The importance of screening for breast cancer cannot be emphasized enough, because early detection can literally be the difference between life and death. Experts recommend that women begin doing regular breast self-exams when they are in their early twenties so they can become familiar with how their breasts feel, which in turn makes it easier to detect any possible changes. Of course, it is never too late to start regular breast self-exams. It is best to do an exam every month a few days after your period ends. If your periods have become highly irregular, try to do your exam the same time each month unless your breasts are swollen and tender.

Instructions on how to do a breast self-exam can be found online, including video instructions, and you can also get free information from your physician or nurse practitioner, at women's health clinics, in books, or online (see "General Health, Nutrition, and Supplement Resources").

CARPAL TUNNEL SYNDROME
If you experience numbness or tingling in your hand or wrist, or a stabbing pain shoots up your arm from your wrist, you may have carpal tunnel syndrome. The carpal tunnel is a narrow passageway at the base of the hands that houses nine tendons and the median nerve, which runs from the forearm into the hand. If this nerve is irritated, injured, or compressed at the wrist, you may experience the symptoms we just described. You may also experience weakness in your hands, causing you to drop objects, or have a constant loss of feeling or the ability to distinguish between cold and hot in one or more fingers. This latter symptom can occur in advanced cases.

Causes/Risk Factors

One of the risk factors for carpal tunnel syndrome is gender: Women are three times more likely than men to develop this condition. Family history of the syndrome is another factor. Certain health conditions, including rheumatoid arthritis, diabetes, obesity, and thyroid problems, and hormonal changes associated with pregnancy, menopause, and hormone therapy may also increase risk.

You may be surprised to learn that computer use has *not* been definitively identified as a risk factor. However, experts believe situations that involve a combination of repetitive, awkward wrist or finger motions, intense pinching or gripping, or working with vibrating tools place people at higher risk for the syndrome.

The bottom line is that carpal tunnel syndrome is often caused by a combination of factors that together increase the pressure on the median nerve and tendons in the carpal tunnel. Some people may have a congenital predisposition for the syndrome by having a small carpal tunnel. Factors that can contribute to development of the syndrome include injury or trauma to the wrist, an overactive pituitary gland, fluid retention related to menopause or pregnancy, a tumor or cyst in the canal, or work stress.

Prevention and Treatment

You can help prevent carpal tunnel syndrome by taking a few precautions. At work or while engaged in activities that involve high-risk motions, such as sewing or woodworking, you can do stretching exercises every forty-five to sixty minutes, take frequent rest breaks, use correct posture and wrist position, and design your work space so your wrist maintains its natural position during your activities. If you hands tend to get cold, keep them warm by wearing fingerless gloves.

A few supplements may help with the inflammation and pain associated with carpal tunnel syndrome.

Best Bets

- *Omega-3 fatty acids.* A dose of 1,000 mg daily of fish oil, which is high in omega-3s, can help reduce inflammation and pain.

- *Boswellia.* Take 1,200 to 1,500 mg of a standardized extract containing 60 to 65 percent boswellic acids two to three times daily for symptom relief.

- *Bromelain.* Take 500 mg (standardized to 2,000 MCU or 1,200 GDU per 1,000 mg) three times daily between meals. If you combine bromelain with boswellia, you enhance the effects of both.

Other Options

- *Vitamin B_6.* Several double-blind studies suggest that vitamin B_6 provides relief. Take 25 mg three to four times daily.

- *Vitamin B_2.* Riboflavin provides relief when taken alone but is even more potent when combined with vitamin B_6. Take 10 mg of B_2 daily.

- *Arnica.* This homeopathic remedy, available in a lotion or cream, can be applied as needed to ease swelling and soreness.

Of Special Interest to Women

The fact that women are three times more likely to have carpal tunnel syndrome has led researchers to speculate that women may have a narrower carpal tunnel. Some experts suggest genetics may play a role, making women more likely to experience musculoskeletal injuries. The major hormone fluctuations that women experience during pregnancy and menopause may cause an accumulation of fluid in the joints, including the wrist, and place women at greater risk of developing the syndrome. In rare cases, women who have had a mastectomy and then develop lymphedema (fluid accumulation) in their arm may get carpal tunnel syndrome due to pressure on the nerve from the edema.

CERVICAL CANCER

Cancer of the cervix—the lower part of the uterus—is typically a slow-developing cancer that begins in the cervical lining. Normal cervical cells gradually undergo precancerous changes, often referred to as cervical intraepithelial neoplasia or dysplasia, that may eventually develop into cancer.

Most women who have precancerous changes of the cervix do not develop cancer. To determine whether such changes are indeed potentially cancerous, doctors can examine samples of the abnormal cells and classify them. When cancer does develop, it usually takes several years, although it can occur in less time. In the United States, cervical cancer accounts for 6 percent of the cancers that affect women; worldwide, it is the second most common cancer in women.

Cervical cancer usually takes one of two forms. Squamous cell carcinoma, which makes up 80 to 90 percent of all cervical cancers, is composed of flat, thin cells. Adenocarcinomas make up 10 to 20 percent of cervical cancers, and these develop from the gland cells in the cervix. Occasionally, cervical cancer has both types of cells and is called mixed carcinoma.

Causes/Risk Factors

The number one risk factor for cervical cancer is infection with human papillomavirus (HPV). More than a hundred viruses are in this group, and some of them can cause cancer of the cervix, especially HPV 16 and HPV 18. Although the presence of HPV is necessary for cervical cancer to develop, most women who have HPV do not get cervical cancer. That means other factors must be involved, and experts speculate that some of the following may play a role:

- Smoking

- Presence of human immunodeficiency virus (HIV) infection

- A diet low in fruits and vegetables

- Being overweight

- History of or current chlamydia infection

- Long-term (five years or longer) use of oral contraceptives

- Multiple pregnancies

- Lack of routine Pap testing

- Family history of cervical cancer

Experts are still not completely sure how certain changes in DNA cause normal cells to become cancerous. Some scientists propose that HPV triggers the production of special proteins that results in the uncontrolled growth of cervical cells, which in some women leads to cancer. Cancer-causing chemicals in cigarettes may damage the DNA of cervical cells and contribute to cancer development, and women who have HIV are very susceptible to cervical cancer.

Prevention and Treatment

Because HPV infection is necessary for development of cervical cancer, preventing this disease is crucial. To avoid HPV, delay having sexual intercourse if you are young, limit your number of sexual partners, avoid having sex with people who have had many sexual partners, and use condoms.

While nutrients and other natural substances cannot cure cervical cancer, some may protect against its development and/or improve quality of life for women who have the disease. Here's what experts have found thus far.

Best Bets

- *B vitamins.* Some studies, including one at the University of Hawaii, suggest that thiamin, riboflavin, folate, and vitamin B_{12} may protect against cervical cancer. Recommended doses are 10 to 100 mg of thiamin, 10 to 50 mg of riboflavin, 400 mcg of folate, and 400 mcg of vitamin B_{12}.

- *Carotenoids.* Alpha-carotene, beta-carotene, lycopene, lutein, and zeaxanthin appear to reduce the risk of cervical cancer, with alpha-carotene offering the most significant protection. A mixed carotenoid supplement is recommended with the following doses: 5,000 IU vitamin A, 1.5 to 1.8 mg alpha-carotene, 3.2 to 3.6 mg beta-carotene, 2 mg lutein, 2 mg lycopene, and 1 mg zeaxanthin.

Other Options

- *Vitamin C.* Women who consume less than 50 percent of the DRI for vitamin C may have ten times the risk of developing cervical cancer. Although a vitamin C deficiency is not common, women with eating disorders or who are on fad diets may be at greater risk. A suggested dose is 500 to 1,000 mg daily in divided doses.

Of Special Interest to Women

The American Cancer Society estimated that about 11,150 cases of invasive cervical cancer would be diagnosed in the United States in 2007, and some experts say that noninvasive cervical cancer is four times more prevalent than the invasive type. Some good news about cervical cancer is that the death rate for the disease declined by 74 percent between 1955 and 1992, largely because of the increased use of Pap testing. This screening technique can detect cell changes before cancer develops and also find early cancer when it is most curable. Thus the importance of undergoing routine Pap testing cannot be emphasized enough. The American Cancer Society recommends the following:

- All women should begin cervical cancer testing about three years after beginning vaginal intercourse, but no later than age 21. A Pap test should be done yearly, or every two years if the liquid-based test is used.

- Beginning at age 30, women who have had normal Pap test results three years in a row may get tested every two to three years, although women with HIV or an otherwise compromised immune system should continue yearly screening. Another option is to get a Pap every three years along with the HPV DNA test.

- Women 70 years and older who have had three or more normal Pap tests in a row and no abnormal results within the last ten years may choose to stop getting tested.

Half of women who are diagnosed with cervical cancer are between 35 and 55 years of age, with slightly more than 20 percent being diagnosed at age 65 or older. Thus it is important for you to continue to screen for this treatable disease for most of your adult life. If you are Hispanic, your risk of developing the disease is more than twice that of non-Hispanic white women, while African American women develop this cancer about 50 percent more often than non-Hispanic white women.

CHLAMYDIA

Chlamydia is the most commonly occurring sexually transmitted disease in the United States. According to the U.S. Department of Health and Human Services, an estimated 2.8 million Americans are diagnosed with chlamydia each year. Because chlamydia usually does not produce symptoms it often goes undiagnosed, but that doesn't mean the problems go away. In fact, about 50 percent of all cases of pelvic inflammatory disease (see "Pelvic Inflammatory Disease"), half of all cases of cervicitis (inflammation of the cervix), and a good percentage of cases of ectopic pregnancy, infertility, urethritis (inflammation of the urethra), and chronic pelvic pain are caused by chlamydia.

The people most likely to develop chlamydia are young, sexually active women who use birth control pills, but any woman who has unprotected sexual relations with an infected male is at high risk of contracting the disease. About 75 percent of infected women have no symptoms, but if they occur, they can include abnormal vaginal discharge and a burning sensation when urinating. If the infection spreads from the cervix to the fallopian tubes, once again symptoms may or may not occur. Women who do experience symptoms may have low back pain, nausea, fever, lower abdominal pain, or bleeding between periods.

Causes/Risk Factors

Risk factors for developing chlamydia include having unprotected sexual relations with a partner whose chlamydia status is not known or having multiple sexual partners. Chlamydia is caused by a bacterium, *Chlamydia trachomatis*, and it can be treated successfully with antibiotics. The disease can be transmitted during genital, anal, or oral sex, even if the person has no signs or symptoms.

Prevention and Treatment

Preventive measures include abstaining from sex, limiting sexual activity to one person who is not infected, and getting tested for the disease if you are sexually active and/or you change partners and/or your partner has had sexual relations with someone else. If you notice symptoms such as an unusual genital sore, burning during urination, or vaginal discharge with odor, stop sexual activity, get tested immediately, and complete treatment, if needed.

Supplements and herbal remedies may help you recover from chlamydia.

Best Bets

• *Probiotics.* If you take antibiotics for chlamydia, take probiotics to help prevent vaginal yeast infections or gastrointestinal disorders that often arise from antibiotic use. If possible, begin taking probiotics before you start antibiotic treatment. Begin with 14 to 16 billion CFUs (colony-forming units) per meal before and while you are on antibiotic therapy, then reduce to 7 to 8 billion CFUs per meal and continue for at least ten days after you end antibiotic treatment.

• *Beta-carotene.* To help maintain healthy mucous membranes and fight infection, take 15,000 IU of beta-carotene two to three times per day for four weeks.

• *Vitamin C.* To enhance your immune system, take 500 mg of vitamin C with bioflavonoids three to four times daily.

Other Options

- *Zinc.* Take this immune system booster during and for two weeks after completing treatment. The suggested dose is 20 mg twice daily. If you take this dose for more than one or two months, also take 1 to 2 mg of copper daily to help maintain a healthy mineral balance.

- *Garlic.* The suggested dose of this natural antibiotic is 600 to 900 mg of dehydrated garlic powder standardized to 1.3 percent allicin in three divided doses per day.

Of Special Interest to Women

Between 5 and 30 percent of pregnant women are infected with chlamydia. Along with the usual complications that all women who have chlamydia can get, pregnant women may experience postpartum endometritis, ectopic pregnancy, preterm labor and delivery, and premature rupture of the membranes. Up to 50 percent of infants born to infected women also have complications, including conjunctivitis (20–50 percent of those exposed) and neonatal pneumonia (10–20 percent). Given the serious risks associated with the combination of pregnancy and chlamydia, all sexually active women should be screened for this disease. The Centers for Disease Control and Prevention recommend yearly testing for all women age 25 and younger, testing for older women based on risk factors (new sex partner, multiple sex partners), and early-first-trimester testing for all pregnant women.

CHRONIC FATIGUE SYNDROME

Imagine feeling too tired to get out of bed, to get dressed, or to walk to the bathroom. Imagine feeling this way every day. If you have chronic fatigue syndrome (CFS), you know what we mean. CFS is a complex disorder in which the main characteristic is extreme fatigue that doesn't improve with sleep. To better define CFS, the International Chronic Fatigue Syndrome Study Group came up with diagnostic criteria. Individuals are considered to have the syndrome if their unexplained persistent fatigue lasts for six months or longer and they have at least four of the following eight primary signs and symptoms:

- Sore throat

- Loss of memory or concentration

- Painful and slightly enlarged lymph nodes in the armpits or neck

- Pain that travels from one joint to another, but without redness or swelling

- Sleep problems

- Unexplained muscle soreness

- Headache that differs from those experienced in the past in terms of severity or pattern

- Extreme exhaustion that lasts more than twenty-four hours after engaging in physical or mental exercise

Approximately 1 million Americans have CFS. More women than men are diagnosed with the syndrome—an estimated four times more—yet experts are not sure whether this is because more women report it or that it truly affects women more frequently.

Causes/Risk Factors

The risk factors and causes of chronic fatigue syndrome are unclear, although there is strong evidence that stress is a major factor. The syndrome also often appears during or shortly after a bout of cold or flu and develops most often in people in their 40s and 50s, but it can occur at any age, even in children. Other risk factors may include a history of eczema, a history of premenstrual syndrome, and panic attacks.

The jury is still out on causes for CFS. Some experts believe an infection is involved, yet no definitive culprits have been identified. Other possible causes may include multiple nutritional deficiencies, food intolerances, thyroid deficiency, and metal and/or chemical sensitivities.

Prevention and Treatment

Since the causes of CFS are uncertain, preventing the syndrome is problematic, but experts generally recommend a nutritious diet, regular exercise, adequate sleep, and managed stress. Several natural supplements may help you manage the disease.

Best Bets

- *Zinc.* Low levels of this mineral in people with CFS suggest that supplementation with 25 to 30 mg daily may provide some benefit.

- *B vitamins.* A London study found that people with CFS improved when taking supplements of the B vitamins thiamin, riboflavin, and pyridoxine. Suggested doses are thiamin, 10 to 100 mg; riboflavin, 10 to 50 mg; and pyridoxine, 25 to 100 mg daily.

- *Coenzyme Q_{10}.* Ninety percent of patients with CFS who took coQ_{10} daily for three months had a reduction or elimination of their symptoms, and 85 percent had an improvement in postexercise fatigue. The suggested dose is 100 mg daily.

Other Options

- *Ginseng.* Use of Asian, American, or Siberian ginseng may relieve fatigue. Suggested doses are 100 mg twice daily of Asian or American ginseng or 2 to 3 g of dried powdered Siberian ginseng.

- *Omega-3 fatty acids.* Omega-3s, specifically EPA (eicosapentaenoic acid), boosted energy levels in people with chronic fatigue, based on a London study. A recommended dose is 1,000 mg daily of an EPA/DHA mix.

Of Special Interest to Women

If you think you have chronic fatigue syndrome, your doctor should conduct tests to rule out *Candida albicans* yeast infection, Epstein-Barr virus, cytomegalovirus, herpes, mononucleosis, and hepatitis, as symptoms of these conditions are similar to those of CFS. Tell your doctor about all your symptoms, including any problems with your menstrual cycle, as these are believed to be risk factors for CFS.

CONSTIPATION

Constipation—the passage of small amounts of dry, hard feces about three times a week or less—is the number one gastrointestinal complaint in the United States. Nearly everyone can expect to experience constipation at some point in their lives, but for about 4.5 million Americans, constipation is chronic. The people most likely to be affected are women, people older than 65, and children.

The strain of constipation can be painful and be accompanied by headache and feeling bloated, uncomfortable, sluggish, or nauseous. Fortunately, for most people these symptoms are temporary and not serious and can be treated successfully at home.

Causes/Risk Factors

Constipation occurs when the colon absorbs too much water or if the colon's muscle contractions (peristalsis) are sluggish or weak, causing the stool to move too slowly through the intestines. This delayed movement results in hard, dry stools. Common reasons for constipation are inadequate fiber and/or fluids in the diet, use of certain medications, abuse of laxatives, inadequate physical activity, ignoring the urge to have a bowel movement, irritable bowel syndrome, changes in routine (e.g., travel, pregnancy, illness), drinking milk, and specific conditions (e.g., stroke, pregnancy, colon cancer).

Prevention and Treatment

If you want to prevent constipation, the best approach is to *not* do many of the items that have been identified as risk factors and causes; that is, eat adequate amounts of fiber (and make sure to balance it with adequate fluid intake), don't abuse laxatives, get enough exercise, and honor the urge to move your bowels. Nondrug treatment of constipation includes the same techniques, but you can complement them with natural supplements.

Best Bets

• *Probiotics.* Beneficial bacteria can eliminate constipation and help maintain a healthy environment in the intestinal tract. Choose a supplement that contains five or more species and take 16 billion CFUs per meal for two to three days. As constipation is relieved, reduce the dose to 10 CFUs per meal for several more days, then 5 CFUs per meal until symptoms resolve.

- *Vitamin C.* For acute constipation, stir 4,000 mg vitamin C powder and 1,500 mg of magnesium oxide powder into 4 ounces of orange juice. Drink it on an empty stomach. One dose is usually sufficient.

- *Flaxseed.* This encourages stool movement. Include 1 tablespoon flaxseed oil daily in food (e.g., on vegetables, in a smoothie) or use 1 to 2 teaspoons of ground flaxseed on cereal, yogurt, or other foods.

Other Options

- *Dandelion.* This mild laxative stimulates the bowel and relieves the discomfort caused by an inflamed bowel. Dandelion contains inulin, a substance that stimulates the growth of probiotics, so it is suggested you use these two supplements together. Suggested doses: 500 mg one to three times daily of powdered root extract (4:1), 100 to 150 drops three times per day of root tincture (1:2) in 45 percent alcohol, or 2 to 8 g three times daily of dried root decoction (tea). (See page 246.)

- *Aloe vera.* Try 0.04 to 0.17 g of dried juice per day to improve bowel movements.

Of Special Interest to Women

If you often experience constipation the week before your period starts, you are not alone: Premenstrual constipation is very common. That's because fluids that normally travel to the colon are retained in other parts of the body, causing you to look and feel bloated. A combination of a slight increase in fiber and water intake plus an additional ten to fifteen minutes of exercise (e.g., brisk walking, yoga, biking) can help relieve symptoms. Constipation is also common during pregnancy due to hormonal changes and abdominal pressure.

Dieting can also cause constipation. Eating stimulates the movement of stool through your intestinal tract. If you tend to eat only one large meal a day and/or you significantly reduce the amount of food you eat, peristalsis becomes weak and sluggish and results in hard stools.

DEPRESSION

It's been called the "common cold of mental illness" because it affects so many people. Approximately 21 million Americans are affected by depression in a given year, according to the National Institute of Mental Health. Nearly twice as many women as men become clinically depressed during their lifetime: that's 10 to 25 percent of women compared with 5 to 12 percent of men.

Depression is more than feeling "blue" or sad; it is a serious condition that impacts the mind and body and every component of a person's lifestyle. There are several types of depression, the more common of which are listed here:

- *Major depressive disorder*, which impairs people's ability to perform everyday activities, such as working, eating, sleeping, and interacting socially. Major depression is often disabling and causes low self-esteem, negative thoughts, and an inability to enjoy activities once found pleasurable.

- *Dysthymic disorder* is a milder yet more chronic type of major depression in which people seem to be mildly depressed all the time and often have been depressed for years.

- *Bipolar disorder*, also known as manic-depression, is characterized by moods that alternate between excitable behavior (mania) and depression. Both of these phases can range from mild to severe in intensity.

• *Seasonal affective disorder* (SAD) typically affects people during the winter months but then dissipates during other months.

A type of depression that specifically affects women is postpartum depression. See "Of Special Interest to Women" on page 52.

Causes/Risk Factors

What makes one person sink into a deep depression after a tragic event and another person go on seemingly unscathed? Answers to such questions—and to what causes depression—are usually not easy to define. The reasons behind a person's depression are highly individual and include genetic factors, lifestyle, family history, and personality. Certain factors can make people more likely to develop depression, including chronic health problems, social isolation (lack of significant social interaction), financial problems, unemployment, marital or relationship problems, loneliness, alcohol or drug abuse, early childhood trauma, or stressful life experiences (e.g., death of a spouse or child, divorce).

Prevention and Treatment

You can prevent depression or its recurrence or keep your symptoms from worsening if you follow a healthy lifestyle: eat nutritious foods, get adequate sleep, exercise regularly, minimize stress, avoid alcohol and drugs, maintain social interactions, and attend to your spiritual well-being. If depression does develop, having a healthy lifestyle in place can speed up your recovery process.

Natural supplements can significantly enhance treatment of depression when used alone or with conventional medical treatment. Consult your doctor before taking any of these natural supplements.

Best Bets

- *St. John's wort.* Studies show St. John's wort to be as effective as selective serotonin reuptake inhibitors (SSRIs) and tricyclic antidepressants in the treatment of mild to moderate depression, and to cause fewer side effects. Suggested doses are 300 to 500 mg (standardized to 0.3 percent hypericin extract) capsules or tablets three times daily with meals, or 40 to 60 drops of liquid extract twice daily.

- *SAM-e.* Use of S-adenosylmethionine (SAM-e) alone and with conventional antidepressant medication results in more effective and faster relief of depressive symptoms, according to several research studies. Effective doses for treatment of depression are 400 to 1,600 mg daily, beginning with 400 mg and gradually increasing the dose over three weeks.

- *5-HTP.* This supplement can relieve depression at doses ranging from 50 to 600 mg daily. Use of 5-HTP has been shown to be equal to or better than standard antidepressant treatment and to be without side effects.

Other Options

- *Valerian.* This herb may reduce anxiety and nervousness. Take any of the following up to three times daily: 150 to 300 mg capsules or tablets, standardized to 0.8 percent valerenic acid; 1 to 2 mL of fluid extract; or 4 to 6 mL of tincture. Take the last dose near bedtime.

- *Omega-3 fatty acids.* Low levels of omega-3s and
  high levels of omega-6s (a common combination in
  the American diet) are associated with depression.
  Taking omega-3 supplements while reducing dietary
  intake of omega-6s (in vegetable oils) can improve
  the balance between these two fatty acids and relieve
  depression. A recommended dose of omega-3s (fish
  oil) is 1,000 mg daily.

- *Folate.* Taking 400 to 800 mcg of folic acid may relieve symptoms of depression and enhance your response to antidepressants if you are taking them.
  Studies show that 15 to 38 percent of people with depression have low levels of folate and that those with
  the lowest levels are the most depressed.

Of Special Interest to Women

About 80 percent of women experience mild depression
after giving birth, which is associated with the sudden decline in hormones that occurs immediately after delivery.
This "blue" feeling usually lasts a few days to two weeks
and then disappears.

But for 10 to 20 percent of new mothers, postpartum
depression is more severe and long-lasting, and it interferes with their ability to care for their new infant. Symptoms typically include anxiety, panic attacks, difficulty
sleeping, lack of interest in their new child, fatigue, poor
concentration, appetite problems, and spontaneous crying.
Some women experience suicidal thoughts and/or thoughts
of harming the infant, although women rarely act on these
thoughts. Postpartum depression is best treated with psychological therapy complemented with natural and/or conventional medical treatment as needed.

DIABETES

An estimated 21 million Americans have diabetes, a metabolic disease in which the pancreas either does not pro-

duce insulin (type 1 diabetes; affects about 5 percent of diabetics) or the insulin it produces is insufficient and/or cannot be used efficiently by the body (type 2 diabetes; occurs in more than 90 percent of diabetics). As a result, an abnormally high amount of sugar (glucose) can accumulate in the bloodstream and cause life-threatening conditions unless treated. A third type of diabetes, gestational diabetes, is discussed in "Of Special Interest to Women."

Approximately 40 million Americans have prediabetes, which means they have many of the risk factors for developing type 2 diabetes. According to the American Diabetes Association, the majority of people with prediabetes will develop the disease within ten years.

Causes/Risk Factors

Risk factors for type 2 diabetes include age greater than 45 years, excess body weight (especially around the waist), a family history of diabetes, high blood pressure (140/90 mmHg or greater), sedentary lifestyle, high-fat diet, high triglycerides (250 mg/dL or greater), high-density lipoprotein (HDL) cholesterol less than 35, impaired glucose tolerance, diabetes during a previous pregnancy, giving birth to a baby weighing more than 9 pounds, and belonging to a certain ethnic group (African Americans, Native Americans, Hispanic Americans, and Japanese Americans have a greater risk than non-Hispanic whites).

Ultimately, type 2 diabetes is caused by a combination of genetic, environmental, and lifestyle factors that contribute to the body's inability to produce enough insulin and/or inability to properly manage the insulin it does produce, resulting in diabetes.

Prevention and Treatment

Preventing diabetes involves avoiding the risk factors over which you have some control, namely, obesity, high blood pressure, high cholesterol and/or triglycerides, lack of exercise, and a high-fat diet. Several natural supplements can help you control blood glucose levels and/or improve insulin resistance. Talk to your doctor before starting any of these supplements.

Best Bets

- *Cinnamon.* Studies show that cinnamon can reduce triglyceride and cholesterol levels and help control blood glucose. Suggested doses are 125 mg of water-soluble extract standardized to 0.95 percent trimeric and tetrameric A-type polymers three times daily, or 3 to 6 g powdered whole cinnamon daily.

- *Magnesium.* Low magnesium levels can make it difficult to control blood glucose levels, and supplementation may improve insulin resistance. Low magnesium levels are also strongly associated with hypertension, obesity, and retinopathy (a complication of diabetes). A dose of 160 mg three times daily is recommended.

- *Chromium.* This mineral reduces insulin resistance and helps reduce the risk of type 2 diabetes. The suggested dose is 600 to 1,000 mg daily in divided doses.

Other Options

- *American Ginseng.* This herb has been shown to improve glucose and insulin control. Suggested dose is 200 mg daily (standardized for 4 percent ginsenosides).

- *Curcumin.* This antioxidant may reduce blood glucose levels and the risk of diabetic complications (e.g., retinopathy, neuropathy). The suggested dose is at least 800 mg daily of extract standardized at 95 percent curcuminoids.

- *Vitamin D plus calcium.* This vitamin/mineral combination can reduce the risk of developing type 2 diabetes and have a positive impact on glucose metabolism. The recommended doses are 1,200 mg of calcium and 800 IU of vitamin D.

Of Special Interest to Women

Between 2 and 7 percent of pregnant women develop diabetes during their pregnancy. Gestational diabetes, one of the most common complications of pregnancy, occurs because the pancreas can't meet the body's increased demand for insulin and so blood glucose levels rise. Once the baby is born, the majority of women with gestational diabetes return to a nondiabetic state. Once a woman has had gestational diabetes, however, she is at greater risk for getting it again during a future pregnancy and for becoming diabetic later in life.

High levels of glucose during pregnancy can cause complications for your baby. If too much glucose gets into the child's blood, your baby may put on extra fat and become too large to enter the birth canal. If you have gestational diabetes, you place your child at greater risk for jaundice, hypocalcemia (low calcium in the blood), compromised heart function, and polycythemia (high number of red blood cells), and place yourself at higher risk for preeclampsia and stillbirth.

DRY EYE SYNDROME

Dry eye syndrome is a chronic lack of moisture and lubrication in the eyes; it can range from mild irritation to severe inflammation. Healthy eyes are constantly protected by a thin tear layer that lubricates and protects the eyes' delicate tissues and helps remove debris. If this layer is not maintained, dry eye develops, with signs and symptoms that may include a scratchy, stinging, or burning sensation in the eyes; a feeling that there is something in your eyes; eye fatigue; sensitivity to light; blurry vision; eye irritation from wind or smoke; and mucus in or around the eyes.

Dry eye syndrome can affect men and women of any age, but it is more common among women after menopause.

Causes/Risk Factors

One obvious cause of dry eye syndrome is environmental: If you live in a windy, dry, dusty climate and/or if your home or office has a dry heating or cooling system, these situations can cause your eyes to be dry. If you spend a lot of time staring at a computer screen, remember to blink often, because insufficient blinking can make your eyes dry. Contact lens users report dry eyes as their number one complaint. People who have rheumatoid arthritis, rosacea, Sjögren's syndrome, or lupus often experience dry eyes as part of their disease.

The natural aging process is a cause of dry eye syndrome, especially during menopause as hormone levels undergo dramatic changes. Some medications, including antihistamines, birth control pills, antidepressants, certain blood pressure medications, and Parkinson's medications, count dry eyes as a side effect. Other causes of dry eye syndrome include a deficiency of the tear-producing glands, eye disease, or eyelids that fail to close completely.

Prevention and Treatment

You can help prevent dry eyes by practicing good eye care:

- Wear glasses when outside to protect your eyes against wind, sun, and flying debris. A wraparound style is best.

- Blink and rest your eyes often, especially if you do visually demanding tasks, such as working at a computer monitor. Several times an hour, take about thirty seconds to close your eyes and then blink rapidly several times to stimulate tear flow.

- Keep the humidity in your home between 30 and 50 percent.

- Use eyedrops as a preventive measure—if you are doing something that is visually challenging, apply drops before your eyes become irritated.

- Stay hydrated. Many people experience some relief simply by drinking more water, especially in drying climates.

Treatment of dry eye syndrome typically includes the preventive measures noted above, as well as use of artificial tears. To these efforts, you can add the following steps.

Best Bets

- *Omega-3 fatty acids.* Omega-3s can reduce the risk of dry eye syndrome and relieve symptoms. Take 1,000 mg of fish oil daily.

- *Flaxseed oil.* This is another source of omega-3 fatty acids, and it has been helpful in relieving dry eye following LASIK eye surgery. Use 1 tablespoon or 3,000 to 6,000 mg as capsules daily.

Other Options

- *Curcumin.* This herb inhibits production of an enzyme that promotes inflammation in the eye. A suggested dose is 400 mg twice daily.

• *Vitamin A/beta-carotene.* Vitamin A is necessary for eye health and specifically the integrity of the mucous membranes and cornea. Although vitamin A deficiency is not common, boosting low levels may benefit those with dry eye. A suggested dose is 5,000 IU of beta-carotene daily.

Of Special Interest to Women

A survey of the nearly 40,000 U.S. women in the Women's Health Study found that dry eye syndrome affects 5.7 percent of women younger than 50 years and 9.8 percent of those 75 years or older. The researchers concluded that the syndrome affects more than 3.2 million American women age 50 and older.

Dry eye is also a symptom of Sjögren's syndrome, an autoimmune disorder in which inflammation causes abnormal dryness of the eyes, mouth, and other areas of the body. Ninety percent of the people with Sjogren's syndrome are women.

ENDOMETRIAL CANCER

Endometrial cancer, also called uterine cancer, is one of the most common cancers among women. This cancer develops in the inner lining of the uterus (the endometrium) and usually grows slowly. Approximately 40,000 women are diagnosed with endometrial cancer each year, and when it is detected early, more than 90 percent of cases can be treated successfully. The disease occurs most often in postmenopausal women, and more often among Caucasians than African Americans.

Causes and Risk Factors

Although the exact cause of endometrial cancer is not known, several factors increase your risk of developing the disease.

- Age 50 or older and being postmenopausal.

- Being overweight.

- Use of estrogen replacement therapy (without progesterone) after menopause. This increases your risk twelvefold.

- Hypertension.

- Diabetes.

- Irregular menstrual periods, which upset the estrogen balance and may increase the risk of getting cancer.

- Early first menstruation, late menopause, or both, which generally means you have had prolonged estrogen exposure, which increases cancer risk.

- Family history of endometrial or other hormone-related cancer.

- Use of tamoxifen, which is used to treat breast cancer. Experts agree, however, that the benefits of tamoxifen outweigh the low risk of endometrial cancer associated with this drug.

Prevention and Treatment

Since the cause of endometrial cancer is not known, early detection is your best defense. The most common sign of endometrial cancer is bleeding or vaginal discharge, which postmenopausal women should immediately bring to the attention of their doctor. Pelvic pain occurs late in the disease.

Natural supplements are meant to complement, not replace, any conventional medical treatments for endometrial cancer. Talk to your doctor about any supplements that you take.

Best Bets

- *Astragalus.* This herb reportedly may activate key cancer-fighting cells—T-cells and natural killer cells. Use the tincture and take 4 to 6 mL in 2 ounces of water three times daily.

- *Green tea.* A type of phytonutrient called polyphenols found in green tea may block estrogen from tumors. Enjoy a cup of green tea three times daily, or take 300 to 400 mg of standardized green tea extract daily.

Other Options

- *Garlic.* Several studies show that a component of garlic, allicin, inhibits the spread of cancer cells. The recommended dose is at least 900 mg daily.

- *Chamomile.* Enjoy a cup of chamomile tea two to three times daily. Chamomile is said to contain chemicals that prevent cancer cells from attaching to new locations.

Of Special Interest to Women

According to the *Journal of the National Cancer Institute,* certain dietary phytoestrogens—specifically isoflavones, coumestans, and lignans—may have a significant effect on your risk of endometrial cancer. Phytoestrogens, which are weak estrogens found in plants, may have anti-estrogenic effects. Researchers studied 500 women ages 35 to 79 who had been diagnosed with endometrial cancer and compared them with 470 healthy women of similar age and ethnicity. Women who consumed the greatest amounts of isoflavones and lignans had a significantly lower risk of endometrial cancer than those who ate the least amount. (Foods with phytoestrogens include soybeans, tofu, miso, and other soy-based items.) The women who got the most benefit were postmenopausal women, while the women most at risk for endometrial cancer were obese women who ate few phytoestrogen-rich foods.

ENDOMETRIOSIS

When the tissue that normally lines the uterus (endometrium) grows elsewhere in the body, the condition is called endometriosis. In most cases, endometriosis occurs on the ovaries, behind the uterus, or on the intestines or bladder, but rarely it appears in other areas, such as the stomach or liver.

Symptoms of endometriosis may include very heavy menstrual flow and pain in the abdomen, pelvis, and lower back. However, some women do not experience symptoms and do not know they have the disease until they have trouble getting pregnant.

Causes/Risk Factors

The cause of endometriosis is unknown; genetics may or may not be a factor. Endometriosis is more likely to occur in women who have never been pregnant. Rarely, a medical condition or infection that affects the pelvic lining and restricts blood flow may contribute to the development of endometriosis.

Prevention and Treatment

Because the cause of endometriosis is unknown, so are ways to prevent it. Treatment typically includes medication to control symptoms and, if necessary, surgery. Various supplements have been effective in relieving symptoms.

Best Bets

- *B vitamins.* Susan Lark, MD, an authority on women's health and the author of *Premenstrual Syndrome Self-Help Book,* recommends taking 50 to 100 mg of a B-complex supplement plus 300 mg of vitamin B$_6$ to manage cramps and inflammation and to regulate estrogen levels.

- *Calcium and magnesium.* To relax the muscles, Dr. Lark also recommends taking 400 to 750 mg magnesium (split into two doses) and 800 to 1,500 calcium (split into three doses) daily, and separate the doses by two hours.

- *Chaste tree berry.* This herb can help restore hormone balance and relieve cramping. A typical dose is 225 mg of the extract three times daily.

Other Options

- *Iron.* If you experience heavy bleeding, get tested for iron deficiency. If you are iron-deficient, take 25 mg iron with 30 mg vitamin C, or higher doses if prescribed by your doctor.

- *Vitamin E.* A dose of 400 to 800 IU daily may relieve cramping and pain.

- *Flaxseed oil.* Just 1 tablespoon in the morning may help relieve cramps and bloating.

FIBROCYSTIC BREAST CHANGES

It's about a week before your period and the symptoms have begun: your breasts are lumpy and tender, they ache and feel heavy, and your nipples itch. These are symptoms of fibrocystic breast changes, a condition experienced by more than 60 percent of women. At one time, these fibrocystic breast changes were referred to as a disease and were believed to increase a woman's risk of developing breast cancer. Today, the condition has been renamed to reflect what it really is—common, benign breast changes, and not a disease—and fears that it can develop into breast cancer have been put to rest.

But fibrocystic breast changes do concern many women because they can be very uncomfortable, painful, and disruptive to their lifestyle. Some women experience mild discomfort that comes and goes; others have constant severe pain and develop multiple lumps. The symptoms are relatively the same each month for some women while they fluctuate month to month for others.

Causes/Risk Factors

The causes of fibrocystic breast changes are not completely understood, but they appear to be related to hormonal changes. Women between the ages of 30 and 50 are most affected, and the condition is rare in postmenopausal women. Experts believe family history and diet (use of caffeine, consumption of high-fat foods) may increase the risk of fibrocystic breast changes. Fat, for example, stimulates the production of estrogen, which contributes to the symptoms of fibrocystic breast changes.

Prevention and Treatment

You may prevent or at least reduce the severity of symptoms by eliminating caffeine, especially the week before your period, and limiting your fat intake to 25 percent or less of your diet. Several supplements may help relieve symptoms, although their effectiveness is still being debated by some experts.

Best Bets

- *Chaste tree berry*. This herb can help balance hormone levels, relieve breast tenderness, and alleviate bloating and cramping. A suggested dose is 225 mg of the extract three times daily.

- *Vitamin B$_6$.* This vitamin may reduce breast swelling and help balance hormone levels. A suggested dose is 50 mg two times daily before breast pain and tenderness occur.

- *Beta-carotene*. Susan Lark, MD, recommends taking 25,000 to 50,000 IU of beta-carotene daily for significant pain relief.

Other Options

- *Vitamin E*. Supplementing with 600 IU of this vitamin may help reduce inflammation and balance your hormones.

- *Magnesium*. Taking 400 mg of magnesium daily for about two weeks before your next period may relieve breast pain.

Of Special Interest to Women

One characteristic of fibrocystic breast changes is free-moving lumps that vary in size and texture. Because fibrocystic breasts are often very dense and it is not easy to distinguish benign breast conditions from breast cancer, all breast lumps should be examined by a health care practitioner. Ask your practitioner to help you establish what is normal for you. Once you are armed with this knowledge, you will be better able to detect any changes during your breast self-exam that should be brought to the attention of your doctor.

FIBROMYALGIA

Do you wake up feeling tired and in pain? Do you go to bed at night feeling the same way? Have your doctors told you they can't find anything specific wrong with you, yet you know something isn't right? You may have fibromyalgia.

Fibromyalgia is a chronic condition characterized by overall pain and stiffness, with certain areas of the body being especially painful when pressure is applied to them. Fatigue, irritable bowel syndrome, depression, facial pain, mood swings, numbness or tingling in the hands or feet, restless legs syndrome, anxiety, and heightened sensitivity to light, odors, sound, and touch are also common in fibromyalgia. The condition is an estimated ten times more common in women than in men, and overall it affects 3 to 6 million Americans.

Cause/Risk Factors

The most popular theory about the cause of fibromyalgia is that people with the condition have a lower threshold for pain because their brain is overly sensitive to pain messages. Exactly why this occurs is not known. Other possible causes or triggers include injury to the central nervous system, infection, disturbed sleep patterns, faulty muscle metabolism, hormone changes, and emotional stress. You are more likely to develop fibromyalgia if you have a family history of the disorder, if you have a rheumatic condition such as rheumatoid arthritis or lupus, or if you are a woman.

Prevention and Treatment

It is difficult to prevent a condition when the cause isn't known, but most experts agree that the best approach is to maintain a nutritious diet, get adequate exercise, avoid fatigue, and minimize and manage stress. Medical treatment focuses on symptom relief, and natural supplements can help with this as well.

Best Bets

- *5-HTP.* Studies show 5-HTP may improve sleep, reduce anxiety and pain, and relieve depression in people with fibromyalgia. An effective dose is 100 mg three times daily.

- *SAM-e.* In studies that compared SAM-e with placebo, SAM-e improved pain, depression, morning stiffness, and fatigue. An effective dose is 200 to 400 mg taken twice daily for six weeks.

- *Coenzyme Q_{10}.* Supplementing with coQ$_{10}$ (150 to 400 mg daily) may improve quality of life, relieve muscle pain, improve mood, and reduce fatigue.

Other Options

- *B complex.* The B vitamins may help increase energy and manage stress. Take one high-potency B-complex supplement daily.

- *Carnitine.* This amino acid can help improve energy levels and enhance the body's ability to use fat to make energy. Take 1,000 to 4,000 mg per day in divided doses.

- *Magnesium and calcium.* This combination has helped some people with fibromyalgia but not others. Some practitioners suggest trying it for several months: 300 to 500 mg of magnesium (split into two doses) and 600 to 1,000 mg of calcium (split into two doses) daily. The magnesium may also help sleep and restless legs. Separate the doses of magnesium and calcium by two hours.

Of Special Interest to Women

- Women with fibromyalgia are more likely to experience breast cysts and dysmenorrhea (very painful menstruation).

- Pregnant women with fibromyalgia usually have more severe pregnancy symptoms (e.g., fatigue, stiffness, pain) than pregnant women who don't have fibromyalgia.

- Symptoms of PMS (e.g., headache, back pain, insomnia, abdominal cramping, confusion) tend to be more severe in women who have fibromyalgia.

GALLSTONES

Gallstones are small, stonelike substances that can form in the gallbladder, the pear-shaped organ located below the liver. These stones tend to develop when bile—the liquid in the gallbladder that helps the body digest fats—contains too much cholesterol, salts, or bilirubin, which cause it to harden.

About 80 percent of gallstones are made primarily of hardened cholesterol and are yellow-green in color; the remaining 20 percent are composed of bilirubin. Gallstones can be as small as a grain of sand or as large as a golf ball.

Gallstones may or may not cause symptoms. A gallstone attack can include severe, steady pain in the upper abdomen that lasts from thirty minutes to several hours; pain between the shoulder blades or under the right shoulder; and nausea or vomiting. Other symptoms may include belching, indigestion, and abdominal bloating. If you experience chills, fever, or sweating, you should seek immediate medical attention.

"Silent stones" is the phrase used to describe gallstones that don't cause symptoms. Approximately 60 to 80 percent of people with gallstones have silent stones. Because these stones do not interfere with gallbladder function, they do not require treatment.

Causes/Risk Factors

Cholesterol gallstones develop when there is an excess of cholesterol or bilirubin or an insufficient amount of bile salts, although why these situations occur is not always clear. Stones may also develop when the gallbladder fails to empty completely or often enough. People who have cirrhosis or hereditary blood conditions such as sickle cell anemia tend to get gallstones. Risk factors for gallstones include:

• Being female, especially if you are pregnant or taking birth control pills or hormone replacement therapy. Overall, women ages 20 to 60 are three times more likely to develop gallstones than are men.

• Age older than 60.

• Having diabetes.

• Being overweight or obese.

• Losing a lot of weight quickly.

• Use of cholesterol-lowering drugs.

• Being a Native American or Mexican American.

Prevention and Treatment

To help prevent gallstones, maintain a healthy body weight, exercise regularly, avoid crash diets or severely limited calorie intake (less than 800 calories per day), and choose a low-fat, high-fiber diet that contains many fresh fruits, vegetables, and whole-grain foods. Supplements that may help prevent or dissolve gallstones or relieve symptoms include the following.

Best Bets

- *Vitamin C.* This vitamin can reduce cholesterol levels in bile. Take 1,000 mg three times daily.

- *Taurine.* This amino acid can be used for up to six weeks alone; then add a mixed amino acid supplement to your daily schedule. Taurine dosage is 1,000 mg twice daily for up to three months.

- *Psyllium.* This fiber can help reduce cholesterol in bile. Take 1 tablespoon of powder dissolved in water twice daily.

Other Options

- *Flaxseed oil.* Suggested dose is 1 tablespoon a day in liquid or pill form. You can mix the oil with food.

- *Curcumin.* This turmeric derivative increases the solubility of bile, which may help prevent the formation of gallstones. Do not use curcumin if you already have gallstones. A suggested dose is 800 mg daily of extract standardized at 95 percent curcuminoids.

Of Special Interest to Women

According to Henry Pitt, MD, director of the Johns Hopkins University Gallstone and Biliary Disease Center in Baltimore, estrogen and progesterone may affect the amount of cholesterol in bile and how the gallbladder fills with and empties the bile. Thus these hormones can set the stage for gallstone development.

Other factors that may contribute to gallstone formation include the use of hormone replacement therapy, taking birth control pills, and multiple pregnancies. Gallstones develop in 3 to 12 percent of pregnant women, and the likelihood increases during the second and third trimesters. Approximately 65 percent of women who have gallstones have no symptoms, and their stones are only discovered during a pelvic sonogram during pregnancy.

HAIR LOSS

Once thought to be a problem that mostly affected men, hair loss is becoming an increasingly worrisome concern among women. According to the American Academy of Dermatology, about 30 million women experience hair loss. Women make up 40 percent of the adult population that is losing its hair.

Unlike men, who typically lose their hair on the temple and crown and have the "monk" bald spot toward the back of the head, women tend to lose hair all over the head. Another difference between male and female hair loss is that in men it is usually age-related, whereas in women it can happen at any time.

Causes/Risk Factors

Hair loss in women is referred to as female pattern hair loss. Although much is still not known about hair loss in women, likely causes include excess testosterone or an underlying medical reason, such as excessive weight loss or anorexia, polycystic ovary syndrome, thyroid disorders, nutritional deficiencies (e.g., vitamin A, iron), extreme emotional stress, major surgery, or severe infection. Situations that involve hormonal fluctuations, such as use of birth control pills, pregnancy, and menopause, may also cause hair loss in some women. Genetics clearly play a role as well.

Prevention and Treatment

One way to prevent hair loss is to improve your lifestyle by better managing stress and following a balanced, nutritious diet. Since hormones often play a part, ask your doctor to check your estrogen, testosterone, and progesterone levels. In many cases, hair loss can be reversed if the underlying cause is corrected (e.g., rebalance hormones, treat thyroid disorder). Along with such steps, you may consider the following supplements.

Best Bets

- *MSM.* This sulfur supplement can be helpful because sulfur is a basic component of hair. A dose of 700 mg daily is suggested.

- *Biotin.* This B vitamin has a major role in hair growth. Some experts recommend 2 to 3 mg of biotin daily for women who are losing their hair.

- *Vitamin B_{12}.* A B_{12} deficiency is not unusual in women who are losing their hair, according to Ted Daly, MD, a hair loss expert and clinical professor of dermatology at Nassau University Medical Center. Choose a sublingual B_{12} supplement at 1,000 mcg daily.

Other Options

- *Iron.* Recent studies show that an iron deficiency can result in hair loss. Before you take an iron supplement, have your doctor check your iron levels and then recommend an appropriate dose for you.

- *Vitamin A.* This vitamin can help prevent hair loss by promoting healthy tissue growth around hair follicles and producing healthy oils in the scalp to help prevent brittleness. Take 5,000 IU as beta-carotene daily.

- *Manganese.* This mineral promotes hair growth. Although manganese deficiency is not common, if you are on a strict diet or have a chronic illness, you may have low levels. A supplement of 10 to 15 mg is suggested.

Of Special Interest to Women

"I'm losing hair on my head but growing it on my chin." This is a common lament among menopausal women who are faced with a decline in estrogen in relation to testosterone, leaving them with an excess of the latter. Some experts say one answer to such hair loss is to restore estrogen levels naturally with phytoestrogens. Because controversy still exists as to whether phytoestrogens can cause breast cancer in some women, talk to your doctor before taking a phytoestrogen supplement. Many experts agree, however, that eating a moderate amount of soy foods, which supply phytoestrogens, is safe and even recommended.

HEADACHE/MIGRAINE

"Headache" is a general term used to describe pain that occurs behind the head, above the eyes and ears, or in the back of the upper neck. Headaches can be primary or secondary. Primary headaches are not caused by any other condition and include tension headaches, migraines, and cluster headaches. Secondary headaches are associated with disease. We focus on tension and migraine headaches.

Approximately 90 percent of adults can expect to experience tension headache during their lifetime, making this the most common of all headache types. Migraine headaches are the second most common type of primary headache, affecting approximately 28 million Americans. Both types of headache are more common among women than men. Cluster headaches, which are rare, mainly affect men.

Causes/Risk Factors

Tension headaches are believed to be the body's response to anxiety, stress, and tension, as they usually appear in adulthood. Coupled with this theory is the belief that stress-induced muscular tension in the neck, jaw, face, shoulders, and head can also cause tension headache. This includes muscle contraction related to temporomandibular joint disorder, arthritis, or other degenerative diseases of the neck and/or spine.

Migraine headaches are likely caused by a combination of enlargement of blood vessels, including the temporal artery, which is located just under the skin of the temple, and the release of chemicals from nerves around the artery and other blood vessels, which in turn causes pain, inflammation, and additional enlargement of the artery. Migraine attacks also increase the activity of the sympathetic nervous system, which controls primitive responses to pain and stress. This increased activity also often causes nausea, vomiting, blurry vision, hypersensitivity to light and sound, and diarrhea.

Risk factors for both tension and migraine headaches include being female and having unresolved stress. For migraines, a family history of the condition increases risk. Hormones play a major role in migraines for women (see "Of Special Interest to Women"). Certain foods, odors, weather conditions, and other environmental factors trigger migraines in some people.

Prevention and Treatment

Avoidance and better management of stress is a good preventive step for tension headaches and migraines alike. Preventing migraines may also include avoiding known triggers, getting regular exercise and adequate sleep, and, if your migraines are associated with hormone levels, reducing your exposure to estrogen, especially with birth control pills and hormone replacement therapy.

Various supplements may alleviate symptoms of both tension and migraine headaches. Here are some suggestions.

Best Bets

- *Feverfew.* Many studies report that migraineurs experienced fewer, less intense, and shorter-duration migraines when they took feverfew daily. The suggested dose is 100 to 300 mg up to four times daily, standardized to 0.2 to 0.4 percent parthenolides. If you choose carbon-dioxide-extracted feverfew, the suggested dose is 6.25 mg three times daily for up to sixteen weeks.

- *5-HTP.* Supplements of 5-HTP increase serotonin levels in the brain and have a positive impact on pain, sleep, mood, anxiety, and aggression. Suggested dose: 50 mg one to three times daily.

- *Magnesium.* This mineral may decrease the duration and intensity of a migraine. Combining magnesium with feverfew and riboflavin has also yielded good results. Magnesium does not appear to help people who experience three or more migraines per month unless the migraines are associated with hormone fluctuations. Suggested dose is 250 to 500 mg daily in divided doses.

Other Options

- *Riboflavin.* This B vitamin reduces the frequency and duration of migraines for many people who take it daily. Suggested dose: 400 mg, which may reduce frequency by at least 50 percent.

- *Coenzyme Q$_{10}$.* In a placebo-controlled, double-blind trial, coQ$_{10}$ significantly reduced the frequency and duration of migraines. The effective dose was 100 mg three times daily.

- *Butterbur.* Three double-blind, placebo-controlled trials showed that butterbur effectively reduced the frequency of migraines by more than 50 percent in at least two-thirds of patients. Dose: 50 mg twice daily is suggested.

Of Special Interest to Women

A relationship between hormones and migraines is clear: 60 percent of women who have migraines can relate them to their menstrual cycle, as the headaches typically occur as estrogen levels decline. However, less than 10 percent of women have headaches only when they menstruate. Therefore, although hormones are involved with migraines, they are not the only trigger. While you work with your health care practitioner to resolve any hormone issues, you need to look for other factors that could be contributing to your head pain.

HEART DISEASE

"Heart disease," also known as cardiovascular disease, is a term used to refer to diseases that affect the heart or blood vessels. Heart disease is the number one cause of death of men and women in the world, and it accounts for 40 percent of all deaths in the United States.

One needs a scorecard to keep track of all the different types of heart disease. Here are a few of the more common types.

- *Coronary artery disease.* This leading cause of heart attacks is characterized by obstructed blood flow to the heart. The most common cause of obstruction is atherosclerosis (see "Causes/Risk Factors").

- *Heart attack.* A heart attack, or myocardial infarction, is damage to the heart caused by a loss of blood supply. The most common cause of obstruction is a blood clot that blocks the flow of blood through a coronary artery, which sends blood to the heart.

- *Cardiomyopathy.* This is a general term for diseases of the heart muscle. Some types of cardiomyopathy are inherited, while others occur for unknown reasons. One of the most common types is idiopathic dilated cardiomyopathy, which is an enlarged heart without a known cause.

- *Congenital heart disease.* This type of heart disease develops before birth and includes many different diseases and conditions that affect the heart muscle, valves, or chambers.

- *Valvular heart disease.* This type of disease affects the heart valves. Valvular heart disease can be congenital or acquired later if you have rheumatic fever, connective tissue disorders, or certain infections.

- *Congestive heart failure.* This is a condition in which the heart is unable to pump enough blood for the body's needs. This lack of sufficient blood flow can cause shortness of breath, fatigue, and fluid retention.

- *High blood pressure.* This is the excessive force of blood as it travels through the blood vessels. It may be the most common form of heart disease and it can cause other types, including congestive heart failure and stroke.

- *Stroke.* A stroke occurs when blood flow to the brain is blocked or when a blood vessel in the brain ruptures.

- *Arrhythmias.* When the electrical impulses in the heart are out of synch, causing the heart to beat too fast, too slow, or irregularly, you have an arrhythmia.

Causes/Risk Factors

The causes and risk factors for heart disease fall into two categories: those you can't change, and those you can. In the first category are family history of heart disease, postmenopause, older age, and race (higher risk among African Americans, American Indians, and Mexican Americans than among whites). Factors you can change include smoking, high blood pressure, inactivity, obesity, uncontrolled diabetes, uncontrolled stress, elevated low-density lipoprotein (LDL) levels, and low levels of high-density lipoproteins (HDL). The most common cause of heart disease is atherosclerosis, a disease in which plaque accumulates in the arteries and obstructs blood flow.

Prevention and Treatment

Most of the risk factors that you can change can also prevent or improve atherosclerosis. That means eating a healthy diet, exercising regularly, maintaining a healthy weight, not smoking, and controlling diabetes, stress, and blood pressure are all important preventive measures. Natural supplements can help both prevent and treat heart disease. Although antioxidant supplements (e.g., vitamins A, C, and E), have not proved to be beneficial in protecting against heart disease, many large studies show that a *diet* high in antioxidants *does*. Therefore antioxidant supplements should not take the place of a nutritious diet.

With that in mind, let's look at the supplements that have been shown to help prevent and treat heart disease.

Best Bets

- *Coenzyme* Q_{10}. There is substantial evidence that coQ_{10} is beneficial either alone or in combination with standard therapies for high blood pressure, heart failure, and other types of heart disease. The suggested dose varies based on the heart condition; typical is 100 mg three times daily.

- *Niacin.* This B vitamin can lower cholesterol and triglyceride levels and reduce inflammation. Studies show that niacin improves HDL cholesterol levels better than statin drugs. Because of the potential for serious side effects, however, niacin should be taken only under a doctor's supervision. Doses typically start low and gradually increase to 1.5 to 3 g daily.

- *Hawthorn.* Many studies support the use of this herb for congestive heart failure and other heart conditions. Dose: *Crataegus oxycantha* extract standardized to 1.8 to 2.0 percent vitexin, 450 mg three times daily. Talk to your doctor before using hawthorn.

Other Options

- *Garlic.* Studies show garlic has the potential to reduce cholesterol and high blood pressure, as well as moderate homocysteine levels. Dose: 300 mg three times daily of standardized dried garlic powder in capsules.

- *Omega-3 fatty acids.* These essential fats can reduce triglycerides, the risk of arrhythmias, and the growth of plaque in the arteries. Dose: 0.5 to 1.8 g daily of fish oil (EPA and DHA) is recommended.

- *Lycopene.* A *Journal of Nutrition* study, which used data from the Women's Health Study of more than 40,000 women, reported that women who consumed the highest amount of lycopene had nearly a 30 percent reduced risk of cardiovascular disease compared with women who consumed the least amount. Dose: 20 to 30 mg daily.

Of Special Interest to Women

This fact cannot be repeated too many times: Heart disease is the number one killer of women. It kills more women than the next five causes of death combined, including breast cancer. Although the news about heart disease in men is promising—since 1979, their death rate has declined by 17 percent—in women it has increased slightly. Why?

According to the American Heart Association, the reason could be that more than 90 percent of primary care doctors don't know that heart disease kills more women than men, or that women are less likely than men to receive angioplasties, stents, and other critical tests and treatments. Perhaps it's because men and women don't always respond in the same way to certain drugs and medical devices, yet many experts don't know how safe any specific medication or device may be for women.

Women need to arm themselves with information and work with experts to get the best preventive care and treatment possible. If your physician is reluctant or unwilling to work with you, find a practitioner whom you can trust. Stay informed by following research results and information provided by organizations, institutions, and websites such as the American Heart Association, Mayo Clinic, National Institutes of Health, Centers for Disease Control and Prevention, WebMD Heart Health Center, and the National Coalition for Women with Heart Disease.

HEMORRHOIDS

Gone are the days when the word "hemorrhoids" was whispered or not even spoken out of embarrassment. Although they aren't usually a topic for discussion at cocktail parties, hemorrhoids are finally getting the attention they deserve. Given that more than 10 million Americans have hemorrhoids—and 60 percent of them are women—that's a lot of people needing attention.

Hemorrhoids are swollen, inflamed veins that can develop inside the rectum (internal hemorrhoids) or at the end of the anus (external). When internal hemorrhoids bleed, which can happen if you pass hard feces, there usually is no pain because the rectum does not have pain-sensing nerves. External hemorrhoids bleed if they are scratched or irritated, and they can be extremely painful if clots form inside them and pressure builds up.

Causes/Risk Factors

Hemorrhoids are most often caused by straining to eliminate stool, chronic constipation, or pregnancy. Pregnancy in particular makes you more likely to get hemorrhoids (see "Of Special Interest to Women"). Your chances of developing hemorrhoids increase if you often postpone having a bowel movement, sit on the toilet for a long time (this places strain on the anal area), or tend to sit for long periods of time. Hemorrhoids may also develop related to obesity, anal intercourse, diarrhea, and some liver diseases, while some people seem to inherit a tendency for hemorrhoids. During periods of stress, hemorrhoids may flare.

Prevention and Treatment

The best way to prevent hemorrhoids is to avoid constipation: eat sufficient fiber every day, get enough fluids to accompany the fiber, exercise regularly, and move your bowels as soon as possible after the urge occurs.

Treatment of hemorrhoids typically involves applying soothing lotions, sitting in warm water (a sitz bath), or sitting on an ice pack. Various natural supplements, used alone or with these approaches, can help relieve symptoms.

Best Bets

- *St. John's wort.* Use the topical form of this herb to help reduce pain and inflammation. Apply as needed.

- *Horse chestnut.* The active ingredient in this herb is aescin, which has been proven to reduce inflammation and strengthen vein walls. A suggested dose is 300 mg taken one or two times daily.

Other Options

- *Psyllium.* This natural fiber supplement can prevent constipation and ease hemorrhoid discomfort. Add ½ to 2 teaspoons of psyllium seed to 8 ounces of warm water, mix well, and drink immediately. Begin with the lowest dose and gradually increase over several days until you reach a dose that works best for you.

- *Flaxseed.* Use the seeds whole or ground. Take 1 to 3 tablespoons in 8 ounces of water daily. Begin with the lowest dose and gradually increase over several days.

Of Special Interest to Women

Hemorrhoids are very common among pregnant women, but the good news is that in most cases, they disappear soon after childbirth. One reason they develop is that the expanding uterus places pressure on the veins in the pelvis and causes them to become swollen. Another reason is that constipation, which is common during pregnancy, can cause hemorrhoids. Yet another reason is that progesterone levels increase during pregnancy, and this hormone relaxes the walls of the veins, which allows them to swell.

Some women develop hemorrhoids immediately after childbirth. They may appear if delivery was traumatic, if the baby was big, or if postpartum constipation set in.

HERPES

Herpes, both oral and genital, is a sexually transmitted disease that affects an estimated 45 million people in the United States, according to the Centers for Disease Control and Prevention. The disease is spread only by direct person-to-person contact: you cannot get it from door handles, toilet seats, or handshakes.

Many people who have herpes are unaware they are infected because they experience few or no symptoms. An outbreak of the disease usually begins as an itching or tingling sensation around the genital area, anus, or mouth, after which the area turns red. Blisters then can form and last from one to two weeks. When the blisters break, they can be very painful. People with herpes are contagious from the time the itching starts until the blisters have completely healed, which can take up to four weeks.

Causes/Risk Factors

Herpes is caused by either one of two types of herpes viruses: herpes simplex virus type 1 (HSV-1) or type 2 (HSV-2). The virus enters the body through microscopic breaks in the mucous linings of the vagina, mouth, or genital skin during intimate contact, travels to the nerve roots near the spinal cord, and settles permanently. During an outbreak, the virus travels along the nerve fibers to the site of the original infection and appears as red skin and blisters. Most cases of oral herpes are caused by HSV-1, while most cases of genital herpes are caused by HSV-2.

Anyone who is sexually active is at risk for genital herpes. Twenty-two percent of Americans are infected with HSV-2, with women at greater risk than men (26 percent vs. 18 percent), although men have twice as many recurrent episodes as women. Another risk factor for herpes is having a compromised immune system. Between 68 and 81 percent of people with HIV (the virus that causes AIDS) have HSV-2. Anyone who takes medications that suppress the immune system is also at greater risk for herpes.

Prevention and Treatment

Herpes prevention can be stated in two words: safe sex. That includes abstinence during outbreaks and use of latex condoms at all other times. Current treatment options include medications that can reduce the frequency and duration of outbreaks, and natural remedies that can provide the same benefits.

Best Bets

- *Lysine.* This amino acid can inhibit the activity of the virus and help reduce itching, tingling, redness, pain, and burning. A recommended dose is 500 to 1,000 mg per day to prevent recurrence, 3,000 to 9,000 mg per day to treat an outbreak. A topical form is also available and can help relieve symptoms.

- *Zinc.* Studies show that zinc can reduce the frequency, duration, and intensity of herpes outbreaks. A suggested dose is 22 mg twice daily.

- *Vitamin C with bioflavonoids.* This combination can promote wound healing and the production of collagen. A suggested dose is 1,000 to 2,000 mg daily.

Other Options

- *Vitamin E.* This antioxidant may speed up the healing of the lesions and help boost your immune system. Try 400 IU daily.

- *Aloe vera.* The gel from this succulent plant can help soothe and heal herpes lesions. Apply the gel directly from the plant or use a commercial product. Use as needed, typically three to four times daily. Continue applications until your symptoms have resolved.

Of Special Interest to Women

Many women who have genital herpes don't realize they
have the disease because they experience atypical symptoms that may include mild itching or slight discomfort,
which they dismiss. Women who are under a great deal of
stress, who have an infection, or who take several medications often have a compromised immune system and are at
risk for more frequent and prolonged outbreaks.

Of real concern is the fact that infected women who are
pregnant can pass the disease to their infant. Approximately
22 percent of pregnant women are infected with HSV-2, yet
up to 90 percent of them don't know they have herpes either
because they have no symptoms or they have mild symptoms that they attribute to other vaginal conditions. Infants
born to women who have genital herpes are at risk for brain
infections, seizures, mental retardation, and death. The risk
to infants contracting herpes while in the womb is 30 to 50
percent if the mother experiences her first outbreak of the
disease during the third trimester.

The take-home message here is not only to practice
safe sex but also to be conscientious about prenatal care
and to consult your ob/gyn before engaging in sexual relations during pregnancy.

HIGH BLOOD PRESSURE (HYPERTENSION)

Approximately 75 million Americans have hypertension, a
condition in which the force of the blood against the walls
of the arteries is abnormally high. Blood pressure is reported using two numbers: systolic pressure (the top number) a measurement of pressure when the heart beats and
forces blood out to the body, and diastolic pressure (bottom
number), a measure of pressure when the heart is resting
between beats. According to the American Heart Association, a blood pressure reading of less than 120/80 is normal,
a reading between 120/80 and 139/89 is considered prehy-
pertension, and a figure of 140/90 or greater is considered
high blood pressure.

Causes/Risk Factors

Ninety-five percent of people who have hypertension have essential (or primary) hypertension, which means it is not caused by or associated with an underlying condition, such as kidney disease. Essential hypertension tends to develop gradually over time, and in most cases the cause is unknown. Experts believe that a combination of factors contribute to essential hypertension, including high salt intake, family history of hypertension, smoking, obesity, sedentary lifestyle, advancing age, stress, excessive alcohol use, and race (hypertension is more common among African Americans and typically strikes them at a younger age than among whites).

Prevention and Treatment

Ways to prevent hypertension relate to its risk factors—that is, maintain a healthy weight, do not smoke, exercise regularly, manage stress, follow a low-fat and low-salt diet, and limit alcohol use. Treatment options should begin with the same efforts, with special attention to diet and exercise that can also help you lose weight and alleviate stress. These lifestyle changes can be highly successful at lowering blood pressure. Natural supplements can complement and enhance your lifestyle changes; if medication should become necessary, they can often be used with it as well.

Best Bets

- *Coenzyme Q_{10}.* At various doses (from 60 to 100 mg twice daily), coQ_{10} can significantly lower blood pressure.

- *Hawthorn.* This herb can dilate blood vessels and help lower blood pressure, as has been seen in several studies. Good results have been seen at 300 and 600 mg daily.

• *Taurine.* This amino acid can lower blood pressure at doses of 3 to 6 mg daily.

Other Options

• *Garlic.* The ability of garlic to lower blood pressure is controversial: Some studies show significant results, while others report no benefit. Effective doses have been 500 to 650 mg or 2 to 3 cloves of fresh garlic daily.

• *Omega-3 fatty acids.* Fish oil may moderately reduce high blood pressure. Of the two fatty acids in fish oil, EPA and DHA, the latter is associated with lowering blood pressure. Suggested dose is 3,000 g daily.

• *Calcium and magnesium.* There are conflicting reports on the ability of this combination to reduce high blood pressure. Advocates recommend 800 to 1,500 mg of calcium and 400 to 750 mg of magnesium daily, taken in divided doses. Take calcium and magnesium two hours apart.

Of Special Interest to Women

Women need to pay more attention to their blood pressure. Here's why.

• Although more men than women have hypertension, women are more likely to die of the disease.

• Women who take oral contraceptives are two to three times more likely to have high blood pressure than their peers who don't take the hormones.

• Only about 60 percent of women with hypertension are being treated, and only about a third of them are controlling their blood pressure optimally. Since uncontrolled hypertension is one of the most important causes of heart disease in women, taking steps to control blood pressure is critical.

• A study published in the February 2008 issue of *Hypertension* reported that among more than 28,000 women age 45 and older, the risk of hypertension decreased in women who had a higher intake of low-fat dairy foods and foods rich in vitamin D, did not change among those who took calcium and vitamin D supplements, and increased in those who consumed few dairy or vitamin D foods.

• Hypertension is the most common medical complication of pregnancy, affecting 10 percent of pregnant women. Timely and accurate diagnosis (to differentiate between preexisting hypertension and pregnancy-induced hypertension) followed by treatment is critical for the health of the mother and child.

HYPOTHYROIDISM

Hypothyroidism is a condition in which the thyroid gland, which is located in the throat, produces abnormally low amounts of the thyroid hormones necessary to maintain a healthy metabolism. Approximately 11 million Americans have hypothyroidism, and it is ten times more common in women than in men.

The thyroid gland produces thyroxine (T4) and triiodothyronine (T3), two hormones that regulate metabolism, affect heart rate, control body temperature, and regulate the amount of calcium in the blood. The abnormally low levels of T3 and T4 characteristic of hypothyroidism results in a slowed metabolism, weak muscles, low body temperature, poor digestion, weight gain, joint pain, cold hands and/or feet, difficulty thinking clearly, and slowed heart function.

Causes/Risk Factors

The most common cause of hypothyroidism in the United
States is Hashimoto's thyroiditis, an autoimmune condition in which the thyroid gland is enlarged and loses its
ability to make thyroid hormones. Other causes include
pituitary disease, destruction of the thyroid gland due to
surgery or radiation treatment, or use of certain medications. Risk factors for hypothyroidism include being female and older than 50, family history of an autoimmune
disease, previous treatment with antithyroid medications
or radioactive iodine, radiation to the neck or upper chest,
or previous thyroid surgery.

Prevention and Treatment

Because the vast majority of hypothyroidism is caused by
Hashimoto's thyroiditis, which can't be prevented, you
cannot prevent hypothyroidism. You can, however, detect
it early if you undergo periodic screening, beginning at
age 35 and every five years thereafter, as suggested by the
American Thyroid Association.

Hypothyroidism requires treatment with medication,
but various natural supplements can complement it.

Best Bets

• *Iodine.* Some people with hypothyroidism have low
  iodine levels, and supplementation with organic iodine can help. To determine if you need iodine, paint
  a spot of tincture of iodine on your skin the size of
  a half dollar. The brown stain should last twenty-four
  hours or longer. The faster the body absorbs the iodine, the greater your deficiency. Do not take iodine
  supplements without your doctor's supervision.

• *Vitamin E.* If you take iodine, supplement with 800 to

1,000 IU natural vitamin E, as it helps the body absorb and use the iodine.

Other Options

- *Taurine*. This amino acid helps produce thyroid hormones. Dose: 200 to 1,000 mg daily.

Of Special Interest to Women

Some things you should know about hypothyroidism:

- About 2 percent of women in the United States are diagnosed with hypothyroidism when they are pregnant.

- Six percent of miscarriages are associated with hypothyroidism during pregnancy.

- Twenty percent of women older than 75 have Hashimoto's thyroiditis, the most common cause of hypothyroidism.

INCONTINENCE

More than 13 million people in the United States experience incontinence, the involuntary, accidental release of urine. Incontinence can affect people of any age, male and female, but women experience it twice as often as men. Some cases of incontinence are short-term, typically associated with a urinary tract infection, constipation, or medication use, but we are concerned with chronic incontinence.

There are two main types of chronic incontinence: stress incontinence and urge incontinence. The most common type of bladder control condition in women is stress incontinence, which can occur when you cough, laugh, sneeze, or do anything else that puts pressure on your bladder. Urge incontinence, often called overactive bladder, happens when you have an urgent need to urinate but can't reach a toilet in time. It is common to have both types of incontinence, especially if you are older than 50.

Causes/Risk Factors

Stress and urge incontinence appear to have different causes. Stress incontinence can be caused by childbirth, being overweight, or any condition that can stretch the pelvic floor muscles, which support your bladder. Once these muscles are weakened, the bladder drops down and pushes against the vagina. This makes it difficult to tighten the muscles that constrict the urethra and thus stop the flow of urine. When you laugh, cough, sneeze, or exercise, the extra pressure these activities place on your bladder can cause urine to leak out.

Urge incontinence is caused by overactive bladder muscles that push urine out of the bladder. The cause of an overactive bladder is often not known, but emotional stress, irritation of the bladder, stroke, and Parkinson's disease are likely candidates.

Prevention and Treatment

One of the easiest and most effective ways to prevent, minimize, and treat incontinence is to practice Kegel exercises, which can be learned in minutes from your health practitioner or by following a few written directions. Other exercises to strengthen the pelvic muscles can also be learned from medical professionals (see "General Health, Nutrition, and Supplement Resources"). Practicing stress reduction and regular bathroom habits are also important. Several natural supplements can complement these efforts.

Best Bets

- *Calcium.* Daily supplementation of 500 to 1,000 mg may help muscle and bone support.

- *Magnesium.* Take 200 to 400 mg daily, along with calcium, to help support the pelvic muscles. Take calcium and magnesium supplements two hours apart.

Other Option

- *Butterbur.* This herb relaxes the detrusor muscle, which in turn reduces pressure on the bladder. Study results show that women who were urinating every 30 to 90 minutes were able to increase the intervals to between 90 and 150 minutes after taking butterbur for eight weeks. A suggested dose is 50 to 100 mg twice daily with meals.

Of Special Interest to Women

Many women understand how the stress, strain, stretching, and weakening of muscles associated with pregnancy and childbirth can contribute to and cause urinary incontinence, but did you know that stress incontinence can worsen during the week before your period begins? That's because lower estrogen levels may reduce muscular pressure around the urethra, which increases the chance of urine leakage. The incidence of stress incontinence also increases after menopause.

INFERTILITY

Infertility is the inability to get pregnant after one year of unprotected sex or the inability to carry a pregnancy to term. For conception to be successful, a series of critical steps must occur: an ovary must release a healthy egg, the egg must travel through a fallopian tube toward the uterus, healthy sperm need to fertilize the egg, and that egg must then implant itself in the uterus, where the hormonal environment must be able to support the development of an embryo.

About 12 percent of women in the United States ages 15 to 44 had difficulty getting pregnant or successfully carrying an infant to term in 2002, according to the Centers for Disease Control and Prevention. The fact that successful conception "takes two," as the saying goes, is evident when we look at why infertility is a problem: In about one-third of cases infertility is related to female factors, in one-third it is related to male factors, and in one-third the reason is unknown or it is a combination of male and female factors.

Causes/Risk Factors

The main cause of infertility in women is failure to ovulate or other problems with ovulation, including polycystic ovary syndrome. Less common causes include uterine fibroids, pelvic inflammatory disease, endometriosis, or physical problems with the uterus. Risk factors for infertility in women include age (fertility declines rapidly beginning at age 30 in women), stress, smoking, alcohol use, sexually transmitted diseases, hormonal problems, obesity, being underweight, poor diet, and athletic training.

Because successful conception takes two, we note here that causes of male infertility may include an inability to have and sustain an erection, insufficient sperm, and unhealthy sperm.

Prevention and Treatment

Rather than try to prevent infertility, you can increase your chances of becoming pregnant in several ways:

- Avoid use of alcohol, tobacco, and street drugs.

- Limit use of caffeine (no more than 250 mg daily).

- Monitor medication use. Talk to your doctor about any medications you are taking, as some prescription and over-the-counter drugs can affect fertility.

- Time intercourse to coincide with ovulation.

- Avoid weight extremes, as hormone production is affected by being underweight or overweight.

A natural approach to treatment of infertility may include the following supplements.

Best Bets

- *Chaste tree berry.* This herb has enhanced fertility in clinical studies and may help women who have abnormal menstrual cycles or polycystic ovary syndrome. A suggested dose is 40 drops of concentrated extract in water taken in the morning.

- *Vitamin E.* In a study of couples with fertility issues, vitamin E supplementation significantly increased fertility. The effective dose is 400 IU daily.

- *Folic acid.* This important B vitamin helps prevent birth defects. Take 400 mcg twice daily.

Other Options

- *Vitamin B_6.* This B vitamin may increase fertility in women who have a history of premenstrual syndrome. The suggested dose is 50 to 200 mg daily, taken along with a vitamin B complex to balance the B vitamins.

Of Special Interest to Women

Infertility is a stressful situation, leaving many women
fraught with anxiety and feelings of helplessness, loss of
control, guilt, isolation, and inadequacy. Research shows
that in general, women in infertile couples have more anxiety and distress than their male partners. The outcome of
attempts to become pregnant are greatly influenced by
emotional factors. Therefore it is important for infertile
women to find effective ways to deal with the psychological turmoil they experience not only to facilitate fertility
but for their mental health as well. Cognitive-behavioral
therapy, couples counseling, support groups, and other interventions are recommended.

INSOMNIA

Do you have trouble falling asleep? Once asleep, do you
wake up often? Do you have trouble falling back asleep
once you wake up? Welcome to the club of about 40
million Americans who suffer with insomnia. Difficulty
falling or staying asleep can be a short-term, on-and-off,
or chronic problem (occurring at least three nights a
week for more than a month). Insomnia can lead to
many complications, including difficulty with memory
and concentration, falling asleep while driving or on the
job, increased risk of injury, and a depressed immune
system.

Causes/Risk Factors

Among the main causes of insomnia are anxiety, depression, and stress. Other causes include physical problems
(e.g., pain, breathing problems, hot flashes, gastrointestinal
conditions, headache, diabetes), use of caffeine and/or alcohol, and use of prescription medications (e.g., some antidepressants, decongestants, digestive medications, and/or
thyroid drugs). Having a fight with your mother-in-law? A
2003 study listed "conflicts with relatives" as a risk factor

for insomnia, along with being overworked on the job or at home, having a sick relative, and having a psychiatric problem.

Prevention and Treatment

To help prevent insomnia, you may need to make some lifestyle modifications.

- If you use caffeine, limit your use to before 2:00 P.M.

- Establish and follow a routine: go to bed and get up at the same time, even on weekends.

- Make your sleep environment welcoming: a comfortable comfortable temperature, nonrestrictive clothing.

- Don't go to bed hungry—have a light snack before retiring.

- Avoid naps.

A natural supplement approach to insomnia includes substances that can help relieve physical and emotional stress.

Best Bets

- *Melatonin.* The suggested dosage is 0.3 to 1.0 mg per night thirty minutes before retiring. You should notice improvement within a few days.

- *5-HTP.* If you are experiencing anxiety, 5-HTP may help. Consider taking 100 to 300 mg per night before bedtime.

- *Magnesium.* A dose of 250 mg before bedtime can relieve both muscle and emotional tension.

Other Options

- *Valerian*. This herb can help relieve anxiety and insomnia. An effective dose is 300 to 600 mg of concentrated root extract one hour before bedtime. For
  tea, steep 2 to 3 g in 8 ounces of hot water for ten to
  fifteen minutes.

- *Chamomile*. A cup of chamomile tea before bedtime
  can reduce stress and aid sleep.

Of Special Interest to Women

Why are so many more women than men burdened with
insomnia? Some research suggests that being divorced
or unemployed increase the risk of insomnia among
women. Hormones are likely the biggest culprits, however. Hormonal changes during premenstrual phase, perimenopause, and menopause can cause sleep disturbances
as well as night sweats, hot flashes, and pain that disrupts sleep.

IRRITABLE BOWEL SYNDROME

It has been called the "ABCD" syndrome, which represents the abdominal cramping, bloating, constipation, and
diarrhea that characterize irritable bowel syndrome (IBS).
This syndrome affects about 20 percent of adults in the
United States, making it one of the most common health
problems in the country. Women are about twice as likely
to get IBS than are men.

IBS is a functional disorder, which means the intestinal
tract appears normal but it doesn't function properly. The
symptoms can be mild to distressing and debilitating, but
they are not life-threatening. IBS does not trigger any structural changes in the bowel and does not increase the risk
of colorectal cancer.

Causes/Risk Factors

Experts don't know what causes irritable bowel syndrome, but most of them believe the immune and nervous systems play a role. Some of the theories under investigation are:

- Normal movement of the colon to push substances through the intestinal tract is dysfunctional, although the reason is uncertain.

- The lining of the colon loses its ability to absorb fluids properly, which results in loose stools.

- The colon in individuals with irritable bowel syndrome is hypersensitive to certain foods (i.e., food intolerance or food allergy) that do not bother most people.

- Stress, even low levels, can cause the intestinal muscles to spasm, which can result in constipation, diarrhea, and/or pain. Stress has this impact on the colon because the intestinal walls are lined with nerve cells that communicate with the brain.

- Some research indicates that a bacterial infection may cause the syndrome.

- People with IBS have abnormally low levels of serotonin, a chemical normally found in high concentrations in the gastrointestinal tract. Low serotonin levels may translate into poor bowel movement and sensation, resulting in pain and other symptoms of IBS.

- Hormones appear to play a role in IBS because nearly half of women with IBS report a worsening of their symptoms in association with menstruation.

Many people occasionally experience symptoms of IBS, but women younger than 35 are at greatest risk for developing the syndrome. Genetics and heredity are also believed to increase risk.

Prevention and Treatment

The most successful ways to prevent IBS are to avoid foods that may trigger symptoms and to effectively manage stress, which is a major factor in this syndrome. Medical treatment for IBS focuses on drugs that may alleviate symptoms. Several natural supplements have proven helpful as well.

Best Bets

- *Probiotics.* Beneficial bacteria can help restore a balanced bacterial environment in the intestinal tract and thus effectively treat IBS. A recommended dose is 5 to 10 billion CFUs daily of a supplement that contains several species of lactobacillus and bifidobacterium.

- *Bromelain.* This digestive enzyme can relieve symptoms of IBS. A recommended dose is 30 to 60 mg daily.

- *Psyllium.* This fiber supplement can gently relieve diarrhea and constipation and thus help regulate elimination. Take 5 to 12 g of supplemental fiber with meals daily to relieve symptoms.

Other Options

- *Peppermint.* The essential oils of this antispasmodic herb can relieve gas, diarrhea, vomiting, and nausea and have a numbing effect on the intestinal tract. Brew peppermint tea using 1 to 2 tablespoons of dried peppermint leaves per 8-ounce cup of boiling water. For enteric-coated capsules, take 1 to 2 capsules (0.2 mL of oil per capsule) three times daily.

- *Ginger.* Ginger helps ease muscle spasms in the intestinal tract, improves muscle tone, and prevents vomiting. Take 250 mg daily.

Of Special Interest to Women

The combination of IBS and pregnancy is an interesting one: Some women say their IBS symptoms disappear, while others report that they get much worse. If you have IBS and are pregnant, you may experience different IBS symptoms during pregnancy. It is not uncommon, for example, for women who used to experience constipation to suddenly get diarrhea. Others find that their symptoms change from month to month. These possibilities seem to indicate that hormones play a significant role in IBS.

LUPUS

Lupus, also called systemic lupus erythematosus (SLE), is an autoimmune disease that affects the immune system and causes it to attack healthy cells in the body. Approximately 1.4 million people in the United States have lupus, and 90 percent of them are women. Lupus is three times more common in black women than in white women, and it is also more common in Hispanic, Asian, and Native American women.

Lupus usually develops slowly and has symptoms that come and go. Of the three different types of lupus, the most common one is SLE, which usually develops in people between the age of 15 and 44 years and can affect nearly any part of the body. Some of its symptoms include a "butterfly" rash across the nose and cheeks, mouth sores, muscle pain and stiffness, arthritis, fever, weight loss, depression, hair loss, photosensitivity, fatigue, abdominal pain, headache, memory problems, and paranoia. Discoid lupus erythematosus (DLE) affects the skin only, and a third type is drug-induced lupus.

Causes/Risk Factors

Except for a probable genetic link, the causes of lupus are unknown; a combination of environmental, hormonal, and genetic factors is likely. Possible risk factors include age, race, exposure to mercury and/or silica, exposure to sunlight, and infection with the Epstein-Barr virus.

Prevention and Treatment

Because the cause of lupus is not known, experts don't know how to prevent it. Medical treatment focuses on relieving symptoms, and several natural supplements can provide relief as well.

Best Bets

- *Omega-3 fatty acids.* Several studies, including a recent British placebo-controlled trial, find that omega-3 supplements significantly improve symptoms of lupus. An effective dose is 3 g daily.

- *DHEA.* Low doses (20 to 30 mg daily) of DHEA have improved quality of life for women with lupus, according to several studies.

Other Options

- *Vitamin D.* Because many people with lupus are photosensitive, a deficiency of vitamin D is possible. Supplement with 200 to 400 IU daily.

- *MSM*. To help reduce arthritis pain and connective tissue breakdown, a dose of 3,000 mg twice daily is suggested.

Of Special Interest to Women

If you have lupus and want to become pregnant, experts recommend that you have your disease under control or you be in remission for twelve months before you get pregnant. Choose an obstetrician and hospital that can manage high-risk pregnancies.

One complication that may develop during pregnancy if you have lupus is preeclampsia, which is characterized by a sudden increase in blood pressure, protein in the urine, or both. Preeclampsia is serious and requires emergency treatment. Another complication is the possibility that your infant will have neonatal lupus. Three percent of infants born to mothers with lupus have neonatal lupus.

MENOPAUSE

Menopause is a natural process—not a disease—in which the ovaries cease functioning. The technical definition of menopause is the absence of menstruation for twelve months, which indicates that there is a transition period. "Perimenopause" is often used to describe the transition period and the changes women's bodies go through as the ovaries shut down. "Postmenopause" is the term for the entire period that comes after the last menstrual period. Most women reach menopause between the ages of 45 and 55.

Symptoms of menopause vary from woman to woman but may include irregular vaginal bleeding, hot flashes, night sweats, mood swings, vaginal dryness, sleep disturbances, increased risk of vaginal and urinary tract infections, urinary incontinence, memory problems, fatigue, redistribution of body fat, weight gain, and skin changes, including worsening of acne and wrinkles. The number, severity, and duration of symptoms are highly individual.

Causes/Risk Factors

For most women, menopause is caused by the natural decline and cessation of ovarian function. A small percentage of women experience menopause when their ovaries are surgically removed (oophorectomy) or they have a hysterectomy in which both ovaries are removed. Use of chemotherapy and/or radiation therapy in ovulating women may also result in menopause, either during treatment or in the months after treatment ceases. In about 1 percent of women, a condition called premature ovarian failure results in menopause before age 40.

Prevention and Treatment

Our goal here is to help you prevent and treat menopausal symptoms naturally so your transition is as smooth as possible.

Best Bets

• *Black cohosh.* Research suggests black cohosh significantly reduces night sweats and hot flashes in menopausal women. In one 2007 study, the herb got significantly better results than fluoxetine, a prescription drug often used to treat menopausal symptoms. The suggested dose is 40 mg daily.

• *Flaxseed.* Ground flaxseed can significantly reduce the frequency of hot flashes, according to recent research. In a Mayo Clinic study, the frequency of hot flashes declined by at least 50 percent in women who took 40 g (about 1.5 ounces) of flaxseed daily.

Other Options

• *Calcium, magnesium, and vitamin D.* This combination is recommended to help prevent osteoporosis, although calcium and magnesium may offer some relief from sleep disturbances. Recommended doses include 1,000 to 1,500 mg calcium, 500 to 750 mg magnesium, and 200 to 400 IU vitamin D daily. Calcium and magnesium supplements should be taken two hours apart.

- *Red clover.* Studies show that red clover may provide limited relief from hot flashes. The recommended dose is 400 to 500 mg daily.

Of Special Interest to Women

During menopause, bone density declines more rapidly than in previous years, placing you at increased risk for osteoporosis and fractures. Therefore if you have not done so already, consider supplementing your diet with calcium, magnesium, and vitamin D, and get a bone scan to determine your bone density.

The risk of heart disease and stroke also increases around the time of menopause. Coronary heart disease rates are two to three times higher in postmenopausal women than in women of the same age who have not reached menopause.

MORNING SICKNESS

If morning sickness truly happened only in the morning, millions of women would probably be grateful. As it is, morning sickness (which is technically termed "nausea and vomiting of pregnancy") can occur any time of the day or night. Although it typically begins around the sixth week of pregnancy, queasiness can begin as soon as two weeks after conception. For more than half of pregnant women, morning sickness is one of the first signs they are going to be a mother. The nausea and/or vomiting are usually worst in the morning and ease up as the day continues. By week fourteen of pregnancy, about half of women say their symptoms disappear, while queasiness may stick around for another month or more in the remaining women.

Causes/Risk Factors

Morning sickness may be caused by changes that occur in the body in the early stage of pregnancy. The rapidly rising levels of estrogen, for example, which cause the stomach to empty more slowly, may cause nausea. Another hormone level that increases dramatically during early pregnancy is human chorionic gonadotropin, which is secreted by the fetus. Pregnant women are often extremely sensitive to smells, so certain odors, such as perfumes, cooking foods, or cigarette smoke, can cause them to gag or feel nauseated. Some experts believe that the gastrointestinal tract may be more sensitive during early pregnancy and thus more likely to cause nausea.

You are more likely to experience morning sickness if you:

- Have a history of motion sickness and/or migraine

- Had morning sickness in a previous pregnancy

- Are carrying more than one child

- Have a family history of morning sickness

- Are carrying a girl (according to one study, women with severe nausea and vomiting were 50 percent more likely to be carrying a girl)

Prevention and Treatment

No one has found a way to completely prevent morning sickness, but you can take steps to reduce its impact. For example, avoid foods and smells that trigger nausea, eat small meals throughout the day, don't drink fluids when you eat, consume foods that are cold or at room temperature (they tend to have less odor than hot foods), and nibble on plain crackers before you get out of bed in the morning and throughout the day.

Natural supplements are usually a safe choice over medications, especially because you don't want to take anything that could harm your child. However, talk to your health care provider before taking any supplements.

Best Bets

- *Ginger.* Studies show that powdered ginger can significantly reduce nausea. In one trial, 88 percent of the women who took ginger felt less nauseated, compared with only 28 percent of the women who took a placebo. The suggested dose is 250 mg of powdered ginger (in capsules) three to four times daily.

- *Vitamin B_6.* Several studies show that vitamin B_6 can significantly reduce morning sickness in some women, although no one knows why it works. Take 10 to 25 mg three times daily.

Other Options

- *Peppermint.* Try a cup of peppermint tea or place a drop of peppermint essential oil on a tissue and breathe in the aroma to help stop nausea.
- *Multivitamin.* There is some evidence that taking a multivitamin can decrease nausea and vomiting more than a placebo. Take a high-potency multivitamin daily, preferably along with a vitamin B_6 supplement.

Of Special Interest to Women

In rare cases, morning sickness can escalate into hyperemesis gravidarum, severe nausea and vomiting that can harm you and your child. Hyperemesis during pregnancy can result in dehydration, weight loss, lightheadedness, and fainting. Sometimes hyperemesis is an indication of a multiple pregnancy or, on rare occasions, a thyroid disorder. If you experience severe nausea and vomiting for twenty-four hours or more, you should contact your physician immediately.

OBESITY AND OVERWEIGHT

Despite the popularity of diet books, weight loss plans, and low-calorie foods, obesity and overweight are an epidemic in the United States. Generally, "obesity" means having too much body fat, which differs from being overweight, which means weighing too much. You can be overweight and have much of the extra weight come from muscle, bone, fat, and/or water. In both cases, a person's weight is greater than is considered to be healthy.

More specifically, the Centers for Disease Control and Prevention defines "overweight" as a body mass index (BMI) of 25 to 29.9 and "obesity" as a BMI of 30 or greater. In some cases, however, individuals may have a BMI that identifies them as being overweight even though they do not have excess fat. This sometimes occurs in trained athletes who may have a high degree of muscularity rather than fat, a feature that is seen in men more than in women.

Recent statistics show that 64.5 million women in the United States—62 percent of adult females in the country— are overweight or obese. Of that figure 33.4 percent are obese. One of the biggest concerns about obesity and overweight is that they increase your risk for or contribute to significant health problems, including but not limited to breast cancer, diabetes, endometrial cancer, gallstones, heart disease, hypertension, incontinence, infertility, kidney disease, low back pain, osteoarthritis, rheumatoid arthritis, and stroke. Losing just 5 to 10 percent of your body weight can prevent or delay some of these conditions.

Causes/Risk Factors

In simplest terms, overweight and obesity are the result of an energy imbalance over a long period of time: People consume more calories than they burn. The cause of such an imbalance, however, can be influenced by many factors, such as individual behavior (including diet and exercise habits), environmental factors, genetics, and cultural expectations. Risk factors for obesity and overweight—a family history of obesity, advancing age, and being female—also play a role.

Except for genetics, people have some control over the other causes and risk factors for obesity and overweight and so also have many opportunities to prevent and treat them.

Prevention and Treatment

How can you have control over risk factors such as age, family history, and sex? If one or both of your parents are obese, chances are environment and habits—inactivity, high-calorie foods—play a big role. You can't change your genes, but you can change your impact on them. Age presents a similar challenge: muscle mass decreases with age, which translates into a decrease in metabolism. This decline can be countered by reducing caloric intake and/or increasing exercise. Women also have less muscle mass and tend to burn fewer calories at rest than men do, but this, too, can be tackled by doing exercises that maintain or build muscle and/or reducing caloric intake.

Several natural supplements can help you on your quest to lose weight.

Best Bets

- *5-HTP.* Serotonin levels decline during dieting and can cause binge eating and cravings for carbohydrates. 5-HTP supplements may reduce hunger by boosting serotonin levels. A suggested dose is 50 to 100 mg thirty minutes before meals, which can be increased to 200 to 300 mg if the lower dose is not effective.

- *Psyllium.* This soluble fiber supplement may help you feel full and decrease hunger cravings. Take 1 teaspoon of psyllium dissolved in 6 to 8 ounces of water before each meal.

- *Green tea.* Several studies indicate that green tea extract boosts metabolism, with much of the credit going to the phytonutrient epigallocatechin gallate (EGCG) in green tea. The suggested dose is 250 mg twice daily (capsules that contain 55 percent EGCG).

Other Options

- *Zinc.* This mineral may increase levels of leptin, a substance that decreases appetite. Zinc may also increase lean body mass and stabilize or decrease fat mass. Take 20 mg daily, along with 1 to 2 mg of copper.

Of Special Interest to Women

Being overweight and female presents some challenges. One is the impact of pregnancy and menopause. Both of these conditions are significant factors in the development of obesity, which suggests that fluctuations in hormone levels predispose women to excessive weight gain. Here are a few others.

- Women have a baseline fat-burning rate that is lower than men's, which may contribute to higher fat storage in women.

- Having lower levels of serotonin helps you feel full at lower levels of food intake, and serotonin levels decrease as body mass increases. This decrease in serotonin occurs at a lower body mass in men than in women, however, which means women don't experience that same sense of fullness until they reach a higher body mass index.

- Leptin, a molecule produced by fat cells, has a role in regulating appetite and energy use. Leptin levels are correlated with body mass index, and they are much higher in women than in men. This may be part of the reason why women are more likely than men to become overweight.

- Obese women who gain weight experience greater increases in blood pressure than their male peers.

OSTEOARTHRITIS

Osteoarthritis is a degenerative joint disease and the most common type of arthritis. It can affect any joint in the body, but it most often impacts the hips, hands, knees, and spine. Symptoms of osteoarthritis include swelling, stiffness (especially in early morning), pain that gets worse as affected joints are used, limited mobility, small nodes on the finger joints, and bony swellings.

More than 20 million people in the United States have osteoarthritis, and men and women are nearly equally affected. The disease most often appears when people reach their 50s and 60s.

Causes/Risk Factors

Primary osteoarthritis is caused by wear and tear on the joints, which breaks down cartilage, the rubbery tissue that cushions the bones at the joints. As the cartilage wears away, the bones rub together, causing swelling, pain, and stiffness. Joint degeneration can be caused by advancing age, excessive stress on the joints, or overuse. Secondary osteoarthritis is caused by outside influences, such as trauma or injury, inherited abnormalities, and joint diseases.

Risk factors for osteoarthritis include advancing age, excess weight, genetic factors, knee injuries, weak thigh

muscles, low intake of vitamins C and D, and certain oc-
cupations (e.g., ballet dancers, professional athletes, con-
struction workers).

Prevention and Treatment

To help prevent osteoarthritis, maintain a healthy weight,
since excess weight places significant stress on the joints,
especially the knees. In fact, overweight women are nearly
four times more likely to develop osteoarthritis of the
knees than women of normal weight. Exercise to increase
muscle strength and/or to lose weight also helps prevent
osteoarthritis.

Medical treatment focuses on relieving symptoms
through use of over-the-counter and prescription medications, hot and cold compresses, exercise, losing weight, and
in severe cases, surgery. Natural supplements can help with
relief of pain, inflammation, and stiffness.

Best Bets

- *Glucosamine and chondroitin.* The ability of glucosamine and chondroitin to relieve symptoms of
osteoarthritis, especially of the knees, is well documented. Both the combination of substances and glucosamine alone can relieve pain, improve range of
motion, and reduce swelling without the side effects
of drugs. Glucosamine may also help restore cartilage. Most studies have shown success using 500 mg
of glucosamine sulfate plus 1,200 mg of chondroitin
taken three times daily.

- *Capsaicin.* This hot-pepper derivative, when applied
topically as a cream, provides pain relief within three
to seven days. Apply capsaicin cream containing 0.025
percent capsaicin two or three times daily.

- *SAM-e.* Both short- and long-term studies have shown positive results when treating osteoarthritis of the knee, hip, or spine with SAM-e. A suggested dose is 1,200 mg daily in divided doses.

Other Options

- *Boron.* This mineral helps build healthy bone and alleviates pain. Take 6 mg daily.

- *MSM.* In several studies, MSM relieved pain and improved function in osteoarthritis. In a placebo-controlled, double-blind trial, MSM was helpful in osteoarthritis of the knee. A recommended dose is 3 g twice daily.

- *Curcumin.* Several recent studies (2007) show curcumin can reduce inflammation in osteoarthritis. An effective dose is 400 mg three times daily, taken on an empty stomach. The addition of 1,000 mg of bromelain can enhance the absorption of curcumin.

Of Special Interest to Women

Osteoarthritis of the knees is very common among women, and some experts believe they know one of the contributing factors: high-heeled shoes. D. Casey Kerrigan, MD, of Harvard Medical School, conducted several studies and found that 2½-inch heels place excessive strain on joints, muscles, and tendons in the knees, which can eventually result in osteoarthritis. Both stilettos and wide-heeled shoes cause the strain, and in fact chunky heels may cause even more pressure because women tend to wear them longer. Therefore, to help prevent osteoarthritis of the knees (and low-back pain), avoid wearing heels.

OSTEOPOROSIS

More than 8 million women and 2 million men have osteoporosis, a condition characterized by the loss of bone density, which weakens the bones and makes them more susceptible to fracture. In fact, people with osteoporosis have no symptoms until a fracture occurs. The only other way to know if you have osteoporosis is to undergo X-ray screenings that determine bone density.

Causes/Risk Factors

The main cause of osteoporosis is a lack of specific hormones, especially estrogen in women and androgen in men. When estrogen levels decline in women, as in menopause, bone loss increases dramatically. Other factors that contribute to bone loss include insufficient calcium and vitamin D, sedentary lifestyle, smoking, excessive alcohol consumption, low body weight, family history of osteoporosis, having an eating disorder, genetic factors, thyroid problems, personal history of fracture as an adult, and use of certain medications, including corticosteroids.

It is well known that women are at greater risk for osteoporosis than are men, especially women who are white or Asian, who have a small frame and/or are thin, and who are postmenopausal. The World Health Organization notes that osteoporosis affects 14 percent of women ages 50 to 59, 22 percent of those 60 to 69, 39 percent of those ages 70 to 79, and 70 percent of those 80 and older.

Prevention and Treatment

To prevent osteoporosis, look at the risk factors and take positive steps: get adequate calcium and vitamin D, exercise, don't smoke, maintain a healthy weight, limit alcohol consumption, and talk to your doctor about any medications you are taking. Use of estrogen replacement is controversial, as it has been linked with an increased risk of certain cancers and heart disease. Use of selective estrogen receptor modulators (SERMs), either by prescription or in natural supplements, bypasses the risks associated with estrogen.

Natural supplements can do much to complement all your efforts to promote bone health.

Best Bets

- *Calcium.* The most bioavailable calcium supplement is calcium hydroxyapatite, which is the only form of calcium that stimulates osteoblasts, the bone-building cells. Take 1,000 to 1,500 mg of calcium daily in divided doses.

- *Magnesium.* Take this important bone-promoting mineral at a dose half that of calcium and two hours apart from calcium. A recommended dose is 500 to 750 mg daily in divided doses.

- *Vitamin D.* This vitamin ensures the absorption of calcium. Take 400 to 600 IU daily.

Other Options

- *Boron.* This mineral improves absorption of calcium and helps increase estrogen levels in the bloodstream. A suggested dose is 6 mg daily.

- *Flaxseed.* Flaxseed contains phytoestrogens, which have shown some benefit in protecting against osteoporosis. One tablespoon of ground flaxseeds daily is recommended.

- *Vitamin K.* Bone proteins need vitamin K to synthesize. The DRI for vitamin K is 90 mcg for women, which you can satisfy partially with a high-potency multivitamin.

Of Special Interest to Women

As women age and enter postmenopause, estrogen levels decline and the risk of osteoporosis increases. This fact led many experts to recommend that women take estrogen replacement or hormone replacement (estrogen plus progesterone) therapy. Estrogen helps slow bone loss and may even help women regain bone density. Yet estrogen and hormone replacement therapies come with risks, which were revealed when results of the Women's Health Initiative were released. Those risks include an increased chance of experiencing heart attack, stroke, blood clots, and breast cancer, all associated with use of hormone replacement therapy, and an increased chance of developing uterine and ovarian cancer, associated with estrogen replacement therapy.

A natural alternative to estrogen and hormone replacement therapy may be a group of phytoestrogens called isoflavones, which are in soybeans and soy products. Isoflavones act like estrogen but provide a significantly weaker action that is sufficient to stimulate the bone-building cells called osteoblasts. At the same time, isoflavones—especially daidzein—inhibit the activity of osteoclasts, cells that break down bone. Many experts believe that the weak estrogenic action of isoflavones makes them a safe alternative to hormone replacement therapy for helping prevent osteoporosis as well as heart disease.

OVARIAN CANCER

Ovarian cancer is the fifth most common cancer among women in the United States and accounts for 4 percent of all cancers that occur in women. Ninety percent of ovarian cancers develop in the cells on the surface of the ovaries and are called epithelial cell tumors.

The death rate from ovarian cancer is higher than that of any other cancer among women, mainly because the cancer is difficult to diagnose early; thus it is usually in an advanced stage when it is discovered. Only half of the women who are diagnosed with ovarian cancer survive five years after their diagnosis. More than 50 percent of cases are among women age 63 or older.

Causes/Risk Factors

The cause of ovarian cancer is largely unknown. A genetic link has been found, however, with the BRCA1 and BRCA2 genes, which cause breast cancer. These mutated genes are also responsible for most inherited ovarian cancer. Women with the BRCA1 mutation have a 35 to 70 percent chance of getting ovarian cancer; those with the BRCA2 gene have up to a 30 percent chance.

If we look at the risk factors for ovarian cancer, we can get a clue as to possible causes. Those factors include age greater than 63, obesity, use of fertility drugs for more than one year, use of estrogen after menopause, family history of ovarian, breast, or colorectal cancer, personal history of breast cancer, and a high-fat diet. Factors that reduce the risk include having had a hysterectomy (reduces risk by 33 percent), having had a tubal ligation (reduces risk up to 67 percent), having had children (the risk decreases as the number of children increases), and having used birth control pills.

Prevention and Treatment

Experts don't yet know enough about ovarian cancer to prevent this disease. Studies have shown, however, that women who used oral contraceptives for five years or longer have about a 50 percent lower risk of developing ovarian cancer than women who never took oral contraceptives. Among women who have BRCA1 or BRCA2 mutations, oophorectomy (surgical removal of both ovaries) protects them against ovarian cancer.

Medical treatment of ovarian cancer consists of surgery, chemotherapy, and/or radiation therapy. Natural supplements may help ease symptoms, improve quality of life, and perhaps slow progression of the disease.

Best Bets

- *Selenium.* Women who have the BRCA1 mutation may get some protection against ovarian cancer by taking selenium because the mineral helps stabilize the mutated genes. The dose used in the study was 276 mcg of selenium daily.

- *Vitamin C.* Experts know this antioxidant can help prevent free-radical damage, which is associated with cancer. A suggested dose is 500 to 2,000 mg daily in divided doses. Do not exceed 1,000 mg daily while undergoing cancer treatment.

- *Carotenoids.* Results of an Australian study and several others found that carotenoids may reduce the risk of ovarian cancer. Experts have not recommended specific doses, although 6 mg is suggested for beta-carotene. Your best bet is to take a carotenoid complex supplement and to eat at least five servings of fruits and vegetables daily.

Other Options

- *Coenzyme Q_{10}.* This antioxidant may help protect against heart damage related to chemotherapy. Take 90 to 400 mg daily.

- *Ginkgo.* A recent Harvard Medical School study found that elements of ginkgo extract and its components (quercetin and ginkgolides) hinder the spread of cancer. A suggested dose is 120 to 240 mg daily of a supplement standardized to 24 percent ginkgo flavonoid glycosides.

Of Special Interest to Women

Ovarian cancer is difficult to detect in its early stages, as there are no reliable screening tests for the disease. The Pap smear can screen for cervical cancer only. Recent studies have found that early-stage ovarian cancer often has identifiable symptoms, although they are common and can easily be confused with those of other diseases.

In a study published in the *Journal of the American Medical Association* in 2004, researchers found that the early warning symptoms most often reported by women who were later diagnosed with ovarian cancer included increase in abdomen size, fatigue, urinary tract symptoms, pelvic pain, and abdominal pain rather than gynecological complaints (e.g., menstrual disorders, pain during intercourse). The researchers also reported that 94 percent of the women had these symptoms in the year prior to their diagnosis, and that 67 percent had recurring symptoms.

If you experience the symptoms discussed here and they have lasted for two weeks or longer, see your gynecologist for testing. Early detection of ovarian cancer is important because the five-year survival rate for women with disease detected early is 70 to 90 percent, compared with 20 to 30 percent for advanced disease.

PELVIC INFLAMMATORY DISEASE

"Pelvic inflammatory disease" (or "disorder"; PID) is a general term for an infection that affects the pelvic reproductive organs in women, including the vagina, cervix, uterus, ovaries and fallopian tubes. An estimated 1 million women experience an episode of PID each year in the United States, and about 100,000 women become infertile because of the disease. Unfortunately, about two-thirds of cases of PID are not recognized by women and their doctors, mainly because not all women have symptoms, and when symptoms do occur they tend to be vague and to mimic those of other common disorders. Signs and symptoms of PID include lower abdominal pain, fever, a foul-smelling vaginal discharge, painful intercourse, painful urination, irregular menstrual bleeding, and pain in the right upper abdomen (rare).

Causes/Risk Factors

PID is caused by bacteria that travel from the vagina or cervix into the other reproductive organs. The most common bacteria to cause PID are those associated with the sexually transmitted diseases (STDs) gonorrhea and chlamydia. Women most at risk for PID are those who are sexually active and of childbearing age. Women younger than 25 are especially vulnerable because the cervix is not yet fully mature, which increases susceptibility to STDs. Other risk factors for PID include having multiple sex partners or having a sex partner who has more than one sex partner, and douching, which may force bacteria into the upper reproductive organs.

Prevention and Treatment

The surest way to prevent PID is to abstain from sexual intercourse or to be in a monogamous sexual relationship with someone who is STD-free. Use of condoms also helps prevent the transmission of gonorrhea and chlamydia. Frequent testing for STDs and early treatment if an STD is diagnosed can prevent the development of PID.

Treatment of PID includes use of antibiotics, typically two different ones. Natural supplements can be used during and after the antibiotic course.

Best Bets

• *Probiotics.* Begin taking probiotics as soon as you are diagnosed so you can prevent development of a yeast infection from the antibiotics. A suggested dose is 5 to 10 billion CFUs per day during the entire antibiotic treatment period and for at least ten days after treatment ends.

- *MSM*. Provides relief from inflammation. A dose of 3,000 mg twice daily is suggested.

- *Omega-3 fatty acids*. These fats help reduce inflammation and pain. A dose of 1,000 mg of fish oil daily is suggested.

Other Options

- *Green tea*. This antioxidant can help fight the infection naturally. Take 250 to 500 mg of extract daily.

- *Bromelain and turmeric*. The combination of this enzyme and herb reduces inflammation and pain. Three times a day, take 40 mg of bromelain and 500 mg of turmeric.

Of Special Interest to Women

PID that is not treated promptly can cause complications, including permanent damage to your reproductive organs. A common complication is the formation of scar tissue in the fallopian tubes, which can cause infertility. Studies show that infertility occurs in 8 percent of women after a single PID episode and in 40 percent who have had three or more episodes. Ectopic pregnancy (when the fetus forms in the fallopian tubes) is another complication: It is six times more likely to occur in women who have had PID than in those who have not. Scar tissue can last for years and cause chronic pain, which may require surgery.

These are all reasons why it's so important to practice safe sex and to be tested for STDs. You may feel embarrassed about the possibility of having an STD, but detecting it early and treating it to prevent PID are much more important, because untreated PID can dramatically change your life.

PREMENSTRUAL SYNDROME (PMS)

It's a condition few menstruating women escape: premenstrual syndrome, or PMS. The American College of Obstetricians and Gynecologists estimates that 85 percent or more of menstruating women experience at least one PMS symptom related to their menstrual cycle. These symptoms occur in the week or two weeks before menstruation begins and typically resolve once bleeding begins. For most women symptoms are mild to moderate and require little or no treatment. About 3 to 8 percent of menstruating women have a severe form of PMS called premenstrual dysphoric disorder (PMDD).

The list of PMS symptoms is long and wide-ranging, although the more common ones include mood swings, tender breasts, headache, food cravings, depression, irritability, fatigue, backache, crying spells, constipation, diarrhea, and bloating. Symptoms may change in number, duration, and severity from month to month or follow a pattern; every woman experiences PMS differently. PMS is more likely to be a problem in women in their late 20s to early 40s.

Causes/Risk Factors

PMS is caused by fluctuating hormone levels, yet why some women are affected by these changes while others are not, or at least not to the same degree, is not fully understood. Research indicates that women who have had at least one child, who have a family history of depression, or who themselves have a history of a mood disorder are more likely to have PMS. Emotional and/or physical stress does not appear to cause PMS, but it can make it worse.

Prevention and Treatment

The line between prevention and treatment is a bit hazy when it comes to PMS. One reason is that PMS can't be prevented, but you can reduce the impact of symptoms. Lifestyle choices such as avoiding caffeine, practicing stress reduction (e.g., yoga, meditation, deep breathing), getting regular exercise to boost endorphin levels, and eating a wholesome diet that avoids excess fats, salt, sugar, and alcohol can go a long way toward providing relief.

Treatment of PMS can include the methods just named, as well as use of over-the-counter nonsteroidal anti-inflammatory drugs and/or natural supplements, which we explain here.

Best Bets

- *Calcium and vitamin D.* This combination may reduce the risk of PMS as well as relieve its symptoms. A daily dose of 1,500 mg of calcium and 400 IU of vitamin D is suggested.

- *Magnesium.* This mineral can help reduce bloating, mood swings, and breast tenderness. A suggested dose is 750 mg daily in two doses, taken two hours apart from calcium.

- *Chaste tree berry.* Studies indicate that 20 to 40 mg of chaste tree berry daily relieves PMS symptoms. In one study of 1,634 women with PMS, 42 percent reported elimination of symptoms and 51 percent said symptoms were reduced after taking 40 mg of chaste tree berry over a three-month period. Other studies showed success with 20 mg daily.

Other Options

- *Vitamin B₆.* Although research on the use of vitamin B$_6$ for PMS is not always favorable, many anecdotal reports are. Women report improvement in water retention, breast tenderness, headache, bloating, and depression. A suggested dose is 50 mg one or two times daily.

- *Dandelion root.* This diuretic helps relieve bloating and eliminates excess estrogen. Suggested dosing: 2 to 3 teaspoons of ground root and leaf in 8 ounces of water, simmered gently for 10 to 15 minutes. Have 2 to 3 cups daily each of the ten days before your period. If you use the extract (1:1 strength, 45 percent alcohol), take 30 drops in warm water three times daily during the same period.

- *Black cohosh.* A popular herb for relief of tension, cramps, mood swings, and water retention. Dose: 250 mg daily, or as directed by your health care professional

Of Special Interest to Women

Dietary changes can have a significant impact on PMS symptoms. Michael Murray, ND, author of *The Encyclopedia of Healing Foods,* notes that reducing or eliminating animal products from your diet, increasing your intake of fiber-rich plant foods, reducing or eliminating salt, and avoiding caffeine can all go a long way toward relieving and preventing PMS symptoms. He also recommends eating a moderate amount of soy (e.g., tofu, tempeh, soy yogurt, soy milk) to take advantage of its phytoestrogens. The mild influence of phytoestrogens may help balance hormone levels when estrogen levels are high, as they are in PMS.

RHEUMATOID ARTHRITIS

It started in her right hand—swollen joints that didn't improve, and after several months they began to ache, making it increasingly difficult to open jars or to work on her keyboard. Forty-six-year-old Clarissa has rheumatoid arthritis, an inflammatory form of arthritis in which the lining of the joints (synovium) swells, causing pain and damage. Rheumatoid arthritis affects 3 million Americans and is about three times more common in women than in men. Clarissa falls within the 40-to-60 age group in which the disease generally first appears, although younger and older people are also affected.

In addition to joint pain and swelling, people with rheumatoid arthritis often experience fatigue, morning stiffness that lasts at least thirty minutes, fever, and the formation of bumps under the skin (rheumatoid nodules) in their arms. The disease typically first affects small joints such as those in the hands, wrists, ankles, and feet, and eventually progresses to the hips, knees, shoulders, jaw, and neck. The severity and duration of symptoms often vary, with alternating periods of increased disease activity (flares) followed by less active times and even remission.

Causes/Risk Factors

Rheumatoid arthritis is an autoimmune disease, which means the body attacks and damages healthy tissues. In rheumatoid arthritis, white blood cells, which are supposed to attack invaders such as bacteria, cause the synovium to become inflamed, which in turn stimulates processes that can damage the bone, cartilage, tendons, and ligaments near the joints. Experts don't know why this occurs and believe it is a combination of genetics, lifestyle, and environmental factors, including exposure to toxins or viruses. Risk factors for rheumatoid arthritis include being female, age 40 to 60, smoking, and family history.

Prevention and Treatment

Treatment of rheumatoid arthritis focuses on relieving symptoms and attempting to slow or stop progression of the disease, as there is no cure. Drugs prescribed for these purposes include nonsteroidal anti-inflammatory drugs (NSAIDs), steroids, immunosuppressants, and disease-modifying antirheumatic drugs (DMARDs), among others. The use of natural supplements alone or to complement these medications can be most helpful.

Best Bets

- *Curcumin.* Recent studies show that curcumin can both prevent and relieve inflammation in people who have rheumatoid arthritis. A dose of 400 to 600 mg three times daily is suggested.

- *Omega-3 fatty acids.* Use of omega-3s can reduce morning stiffness, inflammation, joint pain, number of painful joints, and use of NSAIDs, according to recent studies. Take 1,000 mg three times daily.

- *Vitamins B_1 and B_{12}.* If you are taking NSAIDs, use of these two B vitamins can significantly reduce your need for medication, and perhaps eliminate it altogether. Dose: 100 mg of B_1 and 1,000 mcg of B_{12} (sublingual) daily.

Other Options

- *Selenium.* Levels of this mineral are often low in people who have rheumatoid arthritis, and studies suggest supplementing with 100 mcg per day.

- *Boswellia.* This herb can significantly relieve inflammation and pain. A suggested dose is 400 to 800 mg three times daily.

Of Special Interest to Women

About 70 percent of the Americans who have rheumatoid arthritis are women. It's been noted that women often develop this disease when their sex hormones are in flux (e.g., after pregnancy, near menopause, or postmenopause), yet experts have not yet figured out why this occurs. An attempt to find an answer was undertaken by researchers at Brigham and Women's Hospital/Harvard Medical School who looked at the participants in the Nurses' Health Study, which started in 1976. They compared the 674 women who had rheumatoid arthritis with the approximately 104,000 women who did not.

Investigators found that women who breast-fed had a slightly lower risk, those with very irregular menstrual cycles had a higher risk, and those who took postmenopausal hormones or oral contraceptives had no change in risk for the disease. So while these findings support the case for the role of hormones in rheumatoid arthritis, more research is needed to identify whether a definite link exists and what it may mean for prevention and treatment.

SCLERODERMA

Scleroderma is an autoimmune connective-tissue disease in which the immune system attacks the body and causes scar tissue to form on the skin and organs. This scar tissue can thicken and severely affect organ function and mobility. Approximately 300,000 people in the United States have scleroderma, although experts believe there are many misdiagnosed or undiagnosed cases. Women are affected more than men.

Scleroderma can be localized or systemic. Localized scleroderma is usually mild and can either affect underlying tissues (bones, muscles) or appear as yellowish or ivory-colored dry, hard skin anywhere on the body. Systemic scleroderma develops on the skin and the internal organs and is more complicated. About 90 percent of people with systemic scleroderma also have digestive tract problems, two-thirds have kidney problems, more than half have lung problems, and one-third have scar tissue in the heart or other heart-related problems.

Another type of scleroderma is CREST, an acronym that refers to the combination of five signs: calcium deposits in the skin; Raynaud's phenomenon, a condition in which spasms occur in the tiny vessels that supply blood to the fingers, toes, nose, tongue, and ears; esophageal disease, in which the lower two-thirds of the esophagus malfunctions; sclerodactyly, thickening and tightening of the skin of the fingers and toes; and telangiectasias, tiny red areas on the skin that blanch when pressed. People can have one or more of the components of CREST, although up to 90 percent of those with scleroderma experience Raynaud's phenomenon.

Causes/Risk Factors

The cause of scleroderma is not known. However, experts believe that both genetics and environmental factors are involved in causing the overproduction of collagen—the main connective tissue protein in the body—that results in hardened scar tissue. Many people who have scleroderma have a family history of other autoimmune diseases. Also notable is that some people with scleroderma have associated connective tissue disorders, such as rheumatoid arthritis, systemic lupus erythematosus, or polymyositis.

Prevention and Treatment

Experts have not offered ways to prevent scleroderma since no one knows what causes it. Medical treatment may include topical medications for skin issues, as well as use of NSAIDs, DMARDs, immunosuppressants, and other medications to address respiratory, digestive, or circulation problems. Natural supplements can provide symptom relief and also help restore nutritional deficiencies that are often seen in people who have scleroderma.

Best Bets

- *Selenium.* This mineral is often deficient in people with scleroderma and Raynaud's phenomenon. Since low levels of selenium may contribute to irreversible tissue damage, supplementation is recommended at 200 mcg daily.

- *Vitamin C.* Low levels of vitamin C frequently occur in scleroderma. A suggested amount is 1,000 to 2,500 mg daily in divided doses, as tolerated.

- *Omega-3 fatty acids.* These essential oils can help reduce inflammation and relieve symptoms of Raynaud's phenomenon. A suggested dose is 1,400 mg EPA and 1,000 mg DHA daily, in divided doses.

Other Options

- *Bromelain.* To reduce inflammation and aid digestive problems associated with scleroderma, take 500 mg in divided doses, with meals, for digestive problems; 500 to 2,000 mg in divided doses for inflammation.

- *Ginkgo.* This Chinese herb improves blood flow to the hands and feet, which can significantly reduce Raynaud's symptoms. Take 240 mg three times daily.

Of Special Interest to Women

If you have scleroderma, is it safe for you to get pregnant? Yes and no, according to the research. According to Virginia Steen, MD, of Georgetown University in Washington, D.C., women with scleroderma should not try to get pregnant within three years of diagnosis of their disease. That's the period within which complications such as kidney damage and hypertension can develop and seriously complicate a pregnancy. After three years, it is probably safe. That's not to say that you are home free. High blood pressure is always a consideration in scleroderma, and everyone with the disease is urged to carefully monitor their blood pressure, pregnant or not. Women who have Raynaud's phenomenon as part of their scleroderma will likely find that this complication improves during pregnancy, as blood flow increases during that time and helps warm the extremities.

SHINGLES

If you had chicken pox as a child, as an older adult you may be visited by the same virus, only this time it will cause shingles. This "mature" version of chicken pox typically begins as a burning or tingling pain or itch that occurs in one specific location on one side of the body. After a few days or a week, a rash breaks out, consisting of fluid-filled blisters that often appear in a band that spans one side of the trunk around the waist.

Shingles is not life-threatening, but it can be very painful and debilitating. Fortunately, the rash typically heals in one to three weeks and the pain or irritation usually disappears within three to five weeks. In a small percentage of cases the rash leads to postherpetic neuralgia, a condition that causes the skin to stay painful and hypersensitive to touch for months or years after the rash has disappeared.

Causes/Risk Factors

Shingles is caused by the varicella zoster virus, which lies dormant in the nervous system after a case of chicken pox has resolved. Later in life, typically after age 50, something reactivates the virus and it travels along the nerve fibers to the skin, where the virus multiplies and shingles erupts. Possible triggers include fatigue, stress, skin injury, or a weakened immune system. Shingles develops in about 20 percent of people who had chicken pox infection or vaccine earlier in life. The chance of getting shingles increases with age and in people who have a compromised immune system from cancer, HIV, or organ transplants.

Prevention and Treatment

In 2006, the Food and Drug Administration approved a shingles vaccine for people 60 and older who have had chicken pox. The vaccine reportedly reduces the risk of getting shingles by half, and significantly reduces the severity and complications of shingles in people who still get the disease despite having had the vaccine.

Treatment includes use of antiviral drugs, which work against the infection and may also help prevent postherpetic neuralgia. Natural supplements can be used alone or to complement medical treatment.

Best Bets

- *Lysine.* This amino acid inhibits replication of the virus and thus fights the infection. During an outbreak, take 500 to 1,000 mg three times daily.

- *Vitamin B_{12}.* This B vitamin may help insulate the nerves as well as reduce inflammation and speed up healing. Injections can provide the fastest relief, but oral doses of 2,000 mcg daily are helpful until the infection clears.

- *Astragalus.* Take 300 mg capsules three times daily during an outbreak and then for four to six months after the infection clears to help rebuild the immune system.

Other Options

- *Capsaicin.* This derivative of red chili peppers can relieve the pain of shingles, but use it only after your rash or blisters have healed. The cream is available in

0.0.25 and 0.075 percent strengths. Because capsaicin creams can sting and burn when they are first used, start with a weaker formula. Apply a thin layer three to four times daily as long as you have pain.

- *St. John's wort.* The oil of this herb, when applied to unbroken skin, reduces inflammation and relieves pain. Apply three to four times daily.

Of Special Interest to Women

We have two brief warnings to offer here. One, if you have shingles, avoid contact with infants, children, pregnant women, and adults who have never had chicken pox or received the chicken pox vaccine until your blisters are completely dry. Two, if you are pregnant and have never had chicken pox, avoid contact with anyone who has shingles.

TEMPOROMANDIBULAR JOINT SYNDROME

Temporomandibular joint syndrome (TMJ) is a mouthful—in more ways than one. This condition, also known as myofascial pain dysfunction of the jaw, causes frequent pain in the jaw joint (located in front of the ear on each side of the face) that tends to increase when you move your jaw, especially when chewing. Women are four times more likely to develop TMJ, and it most often affects women ages 20 to 40.

Approximately 10 percent of the adult population in the United States has symptoms of TMJ. In addition to jaw pain, symptoms often include clicking, grating, or popping sounds when moving the jaw, an uncomfortable bite, headache, ear pain, and difficulty completely opening the jaw.

Causes/Risk Factors

Do you grind your teeth or find yourself frequently clenching your jaw when you are stressed? These are the most common causes of TMJ, and most people don't even realize they are doing them. Other causes of TMJ include frequently chewing gum or ice, misaligned teeth, poorly fitted dentures, or a mouth injury.

Prevention and Treatment

If your jaw aches when you wake up in the morning, you could be grinding your teeth while you sleep. Your dental professional may prescribe a bite block, which will prevent you from grinding your teeth. A dentist can also tell you if a physical problem with your mouth is causing the pain.

Treatment of TMJ may include anti-inflammatory or muscle-relaxing drugs, stress reduction techniques, use of a bite block, or hot and cold compresses. Many people turn to natural supplements to enhance their efforts.

Best Bets

- *Calcium and magnesium.* This combination can help the jaw muscle relax. Take 250 mg of calcium and 125 mg of magnesium twice daily, two hours apart.

- *Vitamin B_5.* This B vitamin complements the relief offered by calcium and magnesium. Take 200 mg daily.

Other Options

- *Glucosamine.* In some cases, 500 mg of glucosamine sulfate three times daily may reduce pain and help rebuid cartilage in the jaw joint. Chondroitin sulfate (400 mg three times daily) may be added as well.

- *Vitamin C.* Supplementing with 500 mg of vitamin C twice daily may enhance the range of motion in the jaw joint.

Of Special Interest to Women

One reason why more women than men have TMJ may be due to hormones. Researchers studied more than 12,000 women and found that women who were taking hormone replacement therapy were at least 70 percent more likely than non-therapy-users to have TMJ and that women who were taking oral contraceptives were 20 percent more likely to have TMJ.

URINARY TRACT INFECTION

A urinary tract infection (UTI) is an infection that takes hold in the lower portion of the urinary system—the urethra and the bladder—and in some cases spreads to the ureters and kidneys. Women are no strangers to this condition: Half of all women develop a UTI during their lifetimes, and many have repeat episodes.

Most people experience at least one sign or symptom of a UTI while it develops. These can include a persistent, strong urge to urinate, passing small amounts of urine at frequent intervals, a burning sensation when urinating, strong-smelling urine, and blood in the urine. Depending on the specific type of UTI, you may have other symptoms as well.

- *Acute pyelonephritis.* In this type of UTI, the infection has spread to the kidneys and can cause pain in the upper back and flank, high fever, nausea or vomiting, and chills.

- *Cystitis.* The most common type of UTI, characterized by the signs and symptoms given above.

- *Urethritis.* Inflammation or infection of the urethra that causes burning with urination.

Causes/Risk Factors

The most common cause of cystitis is infection by *Escherichia coli* (*E. coli*), a species of bacteria often found in the gastrointestinal tract. These bacteria typically get into the urethra because of improper hygiene (wiping from back to front after a bowel movement), which introduces the bacteria to the urethra, where they multiply rapidly. Cystitis may also develop after sexual intercourse. In fact, women who are more sexually active are at greater risk of developing a UTI because sexual intercourse can irritate the urethra. Other factors that can increase your risk of getting a UTI are diabetes or other chronic conditions that compromise the immune system, pregnancy, use of certain medications (e.g., cortisone, chemotherapy, antibiotics), use of irritating feminine products, and catheters in the bladder.

Prevention and Treatment

Some everyday habits can help you prevent a UTI.

- Wipe from front to back after urination and bowel movements. This prevents the spread of bacteria to the vagina and urethra.

- Drink plenty of fluids, especially water.

- Urinate as soon as possible after sexual intercourse. This is also a great time to have a full glass of water to help flush bacteria from your system.

- Avoid holding your urine whenever you feel the urge. Retaining urine can stimulate infection.

- Avoid using irritating feminine products in the genital area. These include douches, powders, deodorant sprays, and scented cleansing pads.

Treatment of UTIs typically includes antibiotics. It is important to eliminate the bacteria promptly to prevent the infection from spreading to the kidneys, which can be a more serious infection. Nutritional and herbal remedies can be very helpful in eliminating the infection and preventing recurrence.

Best Bets

- *Cranberry.* Both cranberry supplements and unsweetened juice are effective in preventing UTIs. There is less supporting evidence for using cranberry as treatment. Dose: 300 to 400 mg of cranberry extract capsule twice daily, or 8 ounces of unsweetened juice daily.

- *Uva ursi.* To fight infection, have 2 to 3 cups of uva ursi tea daily (2 teaspoons of herb per 8 ounces of hot water) or use the tincture (1 to 2 teaspoons in warm water twice daily).

- *Probiotics.* If you are taking antibiotics, probiotics are essential to prevent yeast infections and/or recurrence of the UTI. If possible, start the probiotics before you begin the antibiotics and continue the probiotics for about two weeks after you complete your treatment. Take 16 billion CFUs per meal of a mixed probiotics supplement for five days, then reduce to 11 billion CFUs per meal for five days, then 5 billion CFUs per meal until symptoms have resolved.

Other Options

- *Beta-carotene.* Enhance your immune system and the health of your mucous membranes with 25,000 to 50,000 IU daily.

- *Vitamin C.* A dose of 250 to 500 mg twice daily can

make your urine acidic, which inhibits the growth of bacteria.

Of Special Interest to Women

If you are pregnant, you are at increased risk for a UTI, especially from weeks 6 through 24. Changes in the urinary tract during pregnancy, including increased pressure on the bladder from the uterus, which can block the drainage of urine from the bladder, can lead to infection. An untreated UTI can lead to a kidney infection, which may cause early labor and low birth weight. Prompt treatment of a UTI—typically with an antibiotic that will not harm your baby—can eliminate these concerns.

VAGINITIS

Just hearing the word "vaginitis" can start some women itching. In fact, intense itching of the vaginal area is the most irritating symptom of vaginitis, a general term for conditions that involve inflammation of the vagina. Other signs and symptoms may include an odorous vaginal discharge that may be thick or greenish, pain on intercourse, light vaginal bleeding, and painful urination. There are many types of vaginitis, but the most common types are bacterial vaginosis, candidiasis (a yeast infection), and atrophic vaginitis. (Chlamydia, a sexually transmitted type of vaginitis, has its own entry.) Each type has its own cause and course of treatment.

The exact number of women who have vaginitis is difficult to identify. We know, however, that approximately 75 percent of women in the United States experience candidiasis during their lifetime, that between 40 and 50 percent have recurring infections, and that 5 to 8 percent experience chronic candida infections.

Causes/Risk Factors

Bacterial vaginosis is caused by an overgrowth of organisms that are normally found in the vagina. This increase creates an imbalance of bacteria that results in the symptoms we have described. Candidiasis is caused by the fungus *Candida albicans,* and atrophic vaginitis usually occurs after menopause as the result of reduced levels of estrogen, which cause the vaginal tissues to become drier and thinner.

Prevention and Treatment

Although the types of vaginitis differ in several ways, some common preventive measures can help ward off all of them. They include keeping the vaginal area dry and clean; avoiding use of douches, deodorant tampons, strong soaps, and irritating feminine cleansing products; cleaning from front to back after a bowel movement; limiting intake of sugar and alcohol; and taking probiotics on a regular basis.

Medical treatment may include antifungal vaginal creams and suppositories, antibiotics, and other prescription drugs. Various natural supplements may be used alone or to complement medical treatment.

Best Bets

- *Probiotics.* Beneficial bacteria can restore a healthy balance of bacteria in the body and eliminate bacterial vaginosis and candidiasis. Begin with 16 billion CFUs per meal for five days, reduce to 11 billion per meal for five more days, then continue with 5.5 billion per meal until symptoms are under control. A maintenance dose of 2 billion CFUs per day of a probiotic supplement that contains at least five species is recommended. Look for supplements that contain at least one of the following: *L. rhamnosus, L. fermentum, L. delbrueckii, L. plantarum.*

- *Garlic*. There are several ways to use this antifungal and antibacterial herb. You can take 2 capsules daily, each containing 2,500 mcg of allicin; enjoy 1 to 2 raw cloves twice a day; or add 1 teaspoon of garlic juice to 2 tablespoons of plain yogurt, soak a tampon in it, and insert into the vagina. Repeat with a fresh tampon every day until symptoms clear.

Other Options

- *Tea tree oil*. This antimicrobial is especially effective against candidiasis when used as a douche. Mix 1½ tablespoons of oil in 1 cup of warm water and douche 1 to 2 times daily until symptoms clear.

- *Biotin*. This vitamin inhibits yeast growth. Take 300 mcg three times daily during the infection and for several days after it has cleared.

Of Special Interest to Women

The high levels of hormones surging through your body during pregnancy make it easy for you to get a yeast infection. Although they may be uncomfortable, these infections rarely travel into the uterus or harm the infant. Intravaginal treatments (e.g., yogurt-soaked tampons or douching with a solution of tea tree oil) are preferable to oral medications, such as fluconazole, during pregnancy.

For women who are pregnant and who have bacterial vaginosis, most doctors recommend treating it because vaginosis increases the risk of premature birth and premature rupture of the membranes.

VARICOSE VEINS

If you are age 50 or older, there's a 50 percent chance you have varicose veins or will develop them during your remaining years. Varicose veins are swollen, often twisted veins that are raised above the surface of the skin, usually on the backs of the calves or on the inside of the leg. (Hemorrhoids are also a type of varicose veins; they are discussed in their own entry.) They can be flesh-colored, blue, or dark purple. Spider veins, which are similar to varicose veins but are smaller, are so called because they look like spiderwebs. They can form on the legs and face and are often red or blue.

Overall, women are more likely than men to develop varicose or spider veins: 50 to 55 percent of women compared with 40 to 45 percent of men. Spider veins usually do not require medical treatment, but varicose veins can cause significant complications if they are neglected.

Causes/Risk Factors

Veins in the legs have valves that function as one-way flaps that prevent blood from flowing backward as it travels up the legs. If these valves weaken, blood can leak back into the veins and accumulate. This accumulated blood causes the veins to enlarge and become varicose. Spider veins can also form in the same way, although sun exposure, heredity, and hormone fluctuations can also cause spider veins.

Being overweight, pregnancy, standing for extended periods of time, crossing the legs, and even gravity (which makes it difficult for blood to travel up the legs to the heart) are risk factors for varicose veins, as they place additional pressure on the valves in the veins and restrict blood flow. Hormonal changes during menopause and use of birth control pills also place women at greater risk for varicose veins and spider veins.

Prevention and Treatment

To help prevent varicose veins, maintain a healthy weight, do not cross your legs when sitting, exercise regularly to improve leg strength and circulation, elevate your legs when resting, avoid sitting or standing for long periods of time, and eat a low-salt, high-fiber diet. To prevent the development of spider veins on the face, wear sunscreen.

Medical treatment of varicose veins involves minimally invasive procedures such as sclerotherapy (injection of a solution that seals the veins) and laser treatments to surgical procedures. Natural supplements can help prevent or minimize varicose and spider veins.

Best Bets

- *Horse chestnut.* Clinical studies show horse chestnut reduces the edema, itching, and pain of venous insufficiency. In one study, for example, all symptoms greatly improved or disappeared in 5,000 patients who were treated for varicose veins with horse chestnut. Suggested dose is 20 to 50 mg daily.

- *Vitamin C.* Joseph Pizzorno Jr., ND, the noted naturopath and president of Bastyr University in Seattle, recommends taking 500 to 3,000 mg of vitamin C plus 100 to 1,000 mg of bioflavonoids daily for varicose veins. Start with a low dose and gradually increase until you reach your tolerance level.

Other Options

- *Vitamin E.* A dose of 200 to 600 IU daily can help prevent blood clots and facilitate blood flow.

- *Ginkgo.* Ginkgo may strengthen the vein walls and help prevent varicose and spider veins. A suggested dose is 40 mg three times daily.

Of Special Interest to Women

Varicose veins and spider veins are very common during pregnancy. Try all the preventive measures outlined above, and also include resting with your legs higher than your head for at least thirty minutes per day. The good news is that varicose veins related to pregnancy usually disappear within three months of delivery. The downside, however, is that varicose veins tend to worsen with each subsequent pregnancy.

PART II
Supplements

VITAMINS AND MINERALS

B VITAMINS
The B-complex family of vitamins consists of the eight essential B vitamins: thiamin, riboflavin, niacin, pantothenic acid, pyridoxine, folate, biotin, and cobalamin. A ninth vitamin, inositol, is also a member but is not always included in B-complex supplements. Most of the B vitamins are involved in energy metabolism, and often three or more members are necessary for a process to work properly. Therefore if just one of the B vitamins is missing or is in very low supply, the process can break down and cause lethargy and fatigue. That's why health-care professionals recommend taking a B-complex supplement, to ensure people get the full range of B vitamins. If you need higher doses of one or more of the B vitamins for special needs, you can add individual supplements.

Benefits of B Vitamins

To better understand how the B vitamins work together, here's an overview of their characteristics.

- Thiamin (or thiamine), previously known as vitamin B_1, plays a role in nervous system and muscle functioning, various enzyme processes, carbohydrate metabolism, and production of hydrochloric acid (necessary for proper digestion).

- Riboflavin (vitamin B_2) is important for the nervous system, energy production, and red blood cell formation. It may reduce chronic fatigue and improve mood and concentration.

- Niacin (B_3) is the common name for two different compounds: nicotinic acid and niacinamide. Niacin has a role in nervous system function and energy metabolism. High doses of nicotinic acid may reduce cholesterol and triglyceride levels. Niacinamide is used to treat diabetes and to relieve arthritis.

- Pantothenic acid (B_5) is essential for chemical reactions that produce energy and those that manufacture essential fats, cholesterol, steroid hormones, melatonin, and hemoglobin.

- Pyridoxine (B_6) has a role in more than a hundred different enzyme systems, most of which involve protein metabolism. This B vitamin also helps synthesize neurotransmitters in the brain, which is why it is recommended to improve mood/depression and nervous system functioning. Vitamin B_6 supplements can help reduce homocysteine levels (a significant risk factor for heart disease and stroke), regulate blood pressure, act as a diuretic, and help in the treatment of acne, eczema, and psoriasis. The active form of the vitamin, pyridoxal-5-phosphate (PLP), is preferred because it does not cause the peripheral neuropathy or GI upset associated with the "regular" form (pyridoxine).

- Biotin helps in the synthesis and metabolism of fatty acids, amino acids, and cholesterol.

- Folate (folic acid) is probably best known for helping prevent birth defects, but it also works with vitamins B_6 and B_{12} to control homocysteine levels.

- Vitamin B_{12} (cobalamin) helps keep red blood cells and nerve cells healthy, and assists in making DNA. Supplementation with B_{12} is sometimes needed by people who are at greater risk of deficiency, including the elderly, people who don't eat animal products, and anyone who has a gastrointestinal disease. Vitamin B_{12} supplements (along with folic acid and B_6) are also needed to regulate homocysteine levels.

- Inositol plays a key role in the health of cell membranes, especially those in the brain, bone marrow, intestines, and eyes. Because cell membranes regulate the contents of cells, this is a critically important function. Inositol promotes hair growth and helps control estrogen levels; it may also help reduce the risk of breast lumps and reduce cholesterol levels.

How to Take B Vitamins

Look for a high-potency B-complex supplement that provides the following amounts of the various components. The DRIs are given in parentheses. When two figures are given, the first is for adult females, the second for adult males.

- Thiamin: 10–100 mg (1.1 and 1.2 mg).

- Riboflavin: 10–50 mg (1.1 and 1.3 mg).

- Niacin: 10–100 mg (14 and 16 mg).

- Pantothenic acid: 25–100 mg (5 mg).

• Vitamin B$_6$: 25–100 mg (1.3–1.5/1.3–1.7 mg).

• Biotin: 100–300 mcg (30 mcg).

• Folate: 400 mcg (400 mcg for both women and men; 500 mcg for breast-feeding women and 600 mcg for pregnant women).

• Vitamin B$_{12}$: 400 mcg (2.4 mcg). A sublingual supplement is the best absorbed.

• Inositol: There is no standard recommended dose for inositol, but 100 mg is suggested. Take an equal amount of choline at the same time you take inositol and a B-complex supplement.

Best Food Sources

• Thiamin: brewer's yeast, lean pork, legumes, nuts, thiamin-enriched cereals, whole grains

• Riboflavin: dairy products, dark green vegetables, liver and other organ meats, enriched cereals, seafood

• Niacin: beef, chicken, fatty fish (e.g., tuna, salmon), milk, peanuts

• Pantothenic acid: avocados, broccoli, chicken, lentils, milk, mushrooms, split peas, sweet potatoes, yogurt

• Vitamin B$_6$: avocados, bananas, carrots, eggs, fish, greens, lentils, oatmeal, peas, poultry, salmon, sweet potatoes, tuna, turkey, wheat germ, whole grains

• Biotin: avocados, brewer's yeast, chicken, egg yolk, liver, raspberries, wheat bran

- Folate: asparagus, garbanzo beans, grapefruit, leafy greens, lentils, lima beans, oranges and orange juice

- Vitamin B_{12}: beef liver, clams, crab, fortified cereals, mussels, salmon, trout, yogurt

- Inositol: brewer's yeast, cabbage, cantaloupe, dark green leafy vegetables, lentils, peanuts, raisins, unrefined molasses, wheat germ

Of Special Interest to Women

Here are some things women should know about B vitamins.

- Vitamin B_6 (25–100 mg daily) can alleviate some PMS symptoms, including breast pain and tenderness, anxiety, and depression.

- Make sure you get at least 400 mcg of folic acid daily before you become pregnant and 600 mcg during pregnancy to help prevent birth defects. If you breastfeed, take 500 mcg daily.

- Estrogen and oral contraceptives can reduce the amount of vitamin B_6 your body absorbs.

- A study of more than 88,000 nurses found that among women who had at least one alcoholic drink per day, those who also took at least 600 mcg daily of folic acid had a 50 percent less risk of developing breast cancer than women who consumed less than 300 mcg of folic acid daily.

- Women who are strict vegetarians and who want to breast-feed should make sure they are not B_{12}-deficient because their infants can quickly develop a vitamin

B_{12} deficiency and suffer permanent neurologic damage.

- An Italian study found that 200 mg of inositol daily regulated ovarian function in women who had polycystic ovary syndrome.

VITAMIN A

Vitamin A is a generic term for a number of related compounds. We focus on one—retinol—which is often called preformed vitamin A because it is in a form readily available for use by the body. Another type of vitamin A is beta-carotene and other carotenoids (a type of phytonutrient), which are called provitamin A because the body converts them into retinol. Retinol is found in animal-based foods, while beta-carotene and other carotenoids are found in plants. We discuss beta-carotene in the "Carotenoids" entry.

Benefits of Vitamin A

Vitamin A is an antioxidant that is often noted for its impact on the eyes: in fact, retinol is transported to the retina, where some of it is stored in retinal pigment cells. An adequate supply of retinol helps prevent a condition known as "night blindness" and promotes overall eye health. Retinol also supports normal cell reproduction, which is critical for preventing precancerous changes in cells. Vitamin A stimulates the immune system and protects the skin and the cells of the urinary, respiratory, and digestive tracts against infection. The formation of bone, growth hormones, and proteinss also owe a great deal to vitamin A.

How to Take Vitamin A Supplements

The Dietary Reference Intake (DRI) for vitamin A for women age 19 and older is 700 mcg of retinol activity equivalents (RAE) (2,333 IU) daily; for pregnant women, 770 mcg (2,567 IU); and for breast-feeding women, 1,300 mcg (4,333 IU). Many vitamin A supplements provide both retinol and beta-carotene, since retinol can cause side effects while beta-carotene does not. Along with the risk of birth defects, for example, high doses of vitamin A (5,000 IU daily) may be associated with an increased risk of osteoporosis in older adults. The Tolerable Upper Intake Level for vitamin A is 3,000 mcg (10,000 IU) for adults, and pregnant women should avoid any supplement that contains more than 1,500 mcg (5,000 IU). Most health practitioners recommend that everyone get vitamin A from beta-carotene rather than retinol.

Vitamin A deficiency is rare in the United States, but if it occurs it can cause night blindness and a reduced ability to fight infection. Excessive vitamin A intake can cause birth defects, liver abnormalities, reduced bone mineral density, and central nervous system disorders, including headache, nausea and vomiting, blurry vision, and dizziness.

Best Food Sources

Among the few good sources of vitamin A are calf's liver, cod liver oil, cow's milk (with added vitamin A), eggs, butter, and fortified breakfast cereals. In comparison, there are many excellent food sources of beta-carotene (see "Carotenoids").

Of Special Interest to Women

Not too much and not too little: That's what women need to remember about vitamin A. High doses are frequently suggested for the treatment of retinitis pigmentosa, acne, and psoriasis, as well as other skin conditions. Yet high doses of vitamin A—as well as a deficiency—can cause birth defects, which is why women of childbearing age should monitor their vitamin A intake. The bottom line: Get your vitamin A from beta-carotene (see "Carotenoids").

VITAMIN C

Vitamin C, or ascorbic acid, is probably the most well-known vitamin. For people young and old, vitamin C has become synonymous with orange juice and the common cold—drink plenty of juice to ward off the sniffles. But vitamin C is about much more than juice and sneezes.

This nutrient is so important to life that the cells of nearly all mammals—except humans, gorillas, and a few others—can make their own vitamin C. Experts can only speculate as to why humans don't manufacture their own vitamin C. They do know, however, that it is water-soluble, which means it is easily excreted from the body and so needs to be replaced on a daily basis. How much do you need? We discuss that on page 149.

Benefits of Vitamin C

The antioxidant properties of vitamin C provide many of this nutrient's benefits, as it protects the body's cells against damage from free radicals. It is a key factor in the formation and maintenance of collagen, a protein that supports and is a component of bone, tendons, cartilage, bone, teeth, and blood vessels. Vitamin C helps keep the skin and gums healthy and protects against the development of cancer, cardiovascular diseases, cataracts, and joint diseases.

Vitamin C is critical for brain function because it helps make the neurotransmitter norepinephrine, which affects mood. When it comes to energy production, vitamin C is necessary for the synthesis of carnitine, which is critical for transporting fat for conversion to energy. The vitamin also may have a role in reducing blood cholesterol levels.

How to Take Vitamin C Supplements

Although vitamin C is one of the most commonly consumed supplements, many experts still do not agree on how much people really need. The official minimum standard, set by the Institute of Medicine, is 75 mg for women and 90 mg for men. But some health professionals, including followers of the "father of vitamin C," Linus Pauling, say that up to 18,000 mg daily may be necessary in some cases. Many adults, however, find that supplements totaling 500 to 1,000 mg daily give them the added protection they want.

Because some people experience loose stools when they take high levels of vitamin C, increase your intake of vitamin C gradually until you reach your desired goal or a level you can tolerate without experiencing side effects. Dosing tolerance is highly individual: Some people have no problems when they take up to 10,000 mg or more daily, while others find that 1,000 mg is their limit.

Dietary supplements usually contain vitamin C in the form of ascorbic acid, which is best absorbed when it is combined with flavonoids. If you tend to experience stomach sensitivity, you may consider taking a buffered form of vitamin C, which usually combine the vitamin with minerals such as magnesium, calcium, or potassium.

A deficiency of vitamin C can result in dry skin and hair, reduced resistance to infection, nosebleeds, bleeding gums, swollen joints, easy bruising, and anemia. Excessive vitamin C can cause diarrhea and stomach pain.

Best Food Sources

Make sure to eat five to nine servings of fruits and vegetables daily—organic when possible—and include leafy greens and raw produce among your selections. Some of your choices should come from this group of excellent sources of vitamin C: asparagus, bell peppers, broccoli, brussels sprouts, cabbage, cantaloupe, cauliflower, chard, grapefruit, kale, kiwi, lemons and limes, mustard and turnip greens, oranges, papaya, parsley, pineapple, raspberries, spinach, strawberries, tomatoes, watermelon, and zucchini.

Of Special Interest to Women

- Use of oral contraceptives or estrogen therapy can reduce your body's supply of vitamin C, so if you are taking these hormones, make sure you get enough vitamin C in your diet and through supplementation.

- A study published in the August 13, 2007, issue of *Archives of Internal Medicine* reported that vitamins C and E taken together can significantly reduce the risk of stroke (by 31 percent) and heart attack (22 percent) in women. The study involved 8,171 women who took 600 IU of vitamin E, 500 mg of vitamin C, plus 50 mg of beta-carotene every other day for more than nine years.

- A study of more than 13,000 volunteers found that women who took vitamin C supplements daily were 34 percent less likely to develop gallbladder disease or gallstones and that women who were deficient in vitamin C had an increased prevalence of gallbladder disease.

- A clear relationship between vitamin C supplementation and bone mineral density in postmenopausal women was noted in a *Journal of Bone Mineral Research* article: Bone mineral density concentrations were approximately 3 percent higher in women who took vitamin C (average daily intake, 745 mg) and were highest in women who also took calcium and estrogen.

VITAMIN D

Often referred to as the "sunshine vitamin" because the body manufactures it when the skin is exposed to the sun's ultraviolet rays, vitamin D is the only vitamin that is also a hormone. After this fat-soluble nutrient is made by the skin or consumed in food, the liver and kidney help to transform it into an active hormone form which in turn provides benefits to the body (see "Benefits of Vitamin D").

Ten to fifteen minutes of exposure to sunlight three times a week is often quoted as being sufficient for the body to make the vitamin D that it needs. This is misleading, however, because not all sun exposure is the same nor is it equally effective. The closer you are to the equator, for example, the better "quality" the sunlight, but cloud cover and the amount of air pollutants also influence the quality of sunlight. Other factors that impact sun exposure effectiveness are areas of the body exposed to sunlight (face, arms, legs, and back are best), use of sunscreen, and amount of skin pigmentation (darker-skinned people need more sun exposure than lighter-skinned people to make sufficient vitamin D).

Benefits of Vitamin D

The liver and kidneys convert the vitamin D in the skin or food into 1,25 dihydroxyvitamin D, the active hormone form that sends messages to the intestines to increase the absorption of calcium and phosphorus and thus help form and maintain strong bones. Vitamin D also promotes the mineralization of bone, the process by which the various components come together to build bone. More functions of vitamin D are to help maintain a healthy immune system, regulate cell growth and diversity, and, as some evidence suggests, protect against depression, insulin resistance, obesity, and some cancers.

How to Take Vitamin D Supplements

The Institute of Medicine has identified the adult minimum requirements for vitamin D to be 200 IU for people up to age 50, 400 IU for people 51 to 70, and 600 IU for people older than 70. Michael Holick, PhD, MD, a noted vitamin D expert, insists the requirement should be 1,000

IU daily in order to maintain health and reduce the risk of certain cancers, type 1 diabetes, multiple sclerosis, inflammation associated with heart disease, and rheumatoid arthritis.

A vitamin D deficiency can cause serious bone disorders: rickets in children and osteomalacia (softening of the bones) in adults, which is accompanied by muscle weakness and bone pain. Vitamin D deficiency can also cause depression, mood swings, reduced immunity, and sleep problems. Too much vitamin D is not a problem if you rely on the sun for your supply, because the body will not produce too much of the vitamin. It is possible, however, to overdose with oral supplements, which can result in nausea, vomiting, weight loss, weakness, constipation, confusion, and heart abnormalities.

Best Food Sources

It can be difficult to get enough vitamin D from your diet unless you eat a lot of dairy and fish, which is why supplementation is recommended. Good dietary sources are fortified foods such as milk, margarine, cereals, and yogurt, as well as sardines, salmon, and tuna.

Of Special Interest to Women

Vitamin D has long been underappreciated concerning its role in bone health, osteoporosis, and fracture. When it comes to your bones, think beyond calcium: Evaluate your vitamin D intake/UV exposure and talk to your doctor about the possible need for a blood test to determine your vitamin D level.

Although research is still preliminary, there is increasing evidence that vitamin D may protect against some types of cancer, especially breast and colorectal cancers. This is all the more reason to make sure you get at least the minimum requirement for vitamin D, if not the 1,000 IU some experts recommend.

VITAMIN E

When you think of vitamin E, think of the number eight because that's how many different compounds are in the vitamin E family. The four tocopherol members and four tocotrienol members each have an alpha-, beta-, gamma-, and delta- component. Of the eight members, alpha-tocopherol is the most common and biologically active form of this fat-soluble vitamin.

Benefits of Vitamin E

Vitamin E is most touted for its antioxidant activities, especially in the eyes, blood cells, muscles, and nervous system, where it helps protect against cell damage from free radicals. Studies show, for example, that vitamin E can lower the risk of heart disease by about 40 percent by reducing the formation of plaque in the arteries and thus prevent the formation of blood clots. Vitamin E may relieve symptoms of rheumatoid arthritis, reduce the risk of macular degeneration and cataracts, and ease symptoms of premenstrual syndrome and fibrocystic breast syndrome. Some evidence points to its ability to protect against the common cold and flu, as well as reduce the risk of breast and bladder cancer.

How to Take Vitamin E Supplements

Tocopherols and tocotrienols are believed to have different effects on the body, which is why many experts recommend taking a supplement that contains a mixture of the two. One of the components of your supplement should be alpha-tocopherol acetate, which is available in both synthetic and natural forms. The synthetic form (labeled "D,L") is about 50 percent less active than the natural ("D") form. The DRI for vitamin E for adults is 22 to 33 IU daily, which equals 15 to 22 mg. The well-known complementary medicine physician Andrew Weil, MD, recommends taking at least 80 mg (120 IU) of a tocopherol/tocotrienol mixture daily. An alternative is 400 IU daily of mixed natural tocopherols.

Best Food Sources

Dietary sources of vitamin E include almonds, broccoli, greens, kiwi, mango, sunflower seed kernels and oil, and wheat germ oil.

Of Special Interest to Women

Vitamin E was associated with a significant reduction in cardiovascular deaths among women in the Women's Health Study, whose results were published in July 2005 in the *Journal of the American Medical Association.* Approximately 40,000 healthy women 45 years and older participated: Half took vitamin E supplements over ten years and half took a placebo. Among all women who took the vitamin, there was a 24 percent reduction in cardiovascular deaths, while among women 65 and older, there was a 26 percent decrease in cardiovascular deaths and heart attacks, but not strokes.

VITAMIN K

It may be the world's least-researched vitamin, but that may be changing. Vitamin K is a fat-soluble vitamin that is essential for making the liver protein that controls blood clotting. It also assists in the conversion of glucose to glycogen, which is necessary for energy production. Recently, however, scientists found that vitamin K plays a role in bone health, a big concern in our aging population.

Natural vitamin K occurs in two forms: phylloquinone (K1), which is found in plants, and menaquinone (K2), which can be synthesized by bacteria in the large intestine. A third form, called menadione (K3), is manmade.

Benefits of Vitamin K

Vitamin K is critical for the functioning of several proteins that are involved in blood clotting. Without vitamin K, you would bleed to death. Another benefit of vitamin K is its role in bone health and the prevention of osteoporosis. Many studies are showing how vitamin K can improve bone mineral density and help decrease the risk of fracture.

How to Take Vitamin K Supplements

The DRI for vitamin K is 120 mcg for males and 90 mcg for females. Vitamin K supplements should be taken only if blood tests reveal a deficiency and you are under a doctor's supervision. In most cases, low blood levels of vitamin K can be remedied by increasing your intake of foods rich in vitamin K. Before you increase your intake of these foods or take a supplement, talk to your doctor if you are also taking anticoagulant medication.

A deficiency of vitamin K can cause internal hemorrhaging, easy bruising, bleeding gums, and nosebleeds in people of all ages. So far, experts have not seen any adverse effects from getting too much natural vitamin K. Because high intake of the synthetic form can cause anemia, jaundice, and other medical problems, the Food and Drug Administration does not allow it to be used in supplements.

Best Food Sources

The best dietary sources of vitamin K are leafy greens (collards, kale, mustard greens, spinach, Swiss chard, turnip greens) followed by asparagus, broccoli, brussels sprouts, cauliflower, celery, green tea, parsley, romaine lettuce, and soybeans.

Of Special Interest to Women

Women who have low blood levels of vitamin K have lower bone mineral density and higher fracture rates than women who have high levels of the vitamin. These findings have been supported by the result of a study of more than 70,000 women, in which investigators found that those who consumed a large amount of vitamin K in their diets had a lower risk of hip fracture. It appears that vitamin K levels decrease with age and the risk of fracture increases. Therefore, older women need to be especially careful to get enough vitamin K.

If you are pregnant, eat foods with high vitamin K content during your pregnancy because the vitamin is transferred to your fetus. If you plan to breast-feed or are already breast-feeding, talk to your doctor about giving your infant vitamin K (formulas contain this supplement) or about taking a supplement yourself for the first three months of breast-feeding to help your child establish a healthy vitamin K level.

BORON

Boron is a trace element concentrated in the bone, thyroid, and spleen. These locations indicate that it is important in bone health and hormone metabolism. Although boron has not received as much attention as other nutrients, researchers have made some interesting observations about this mineral. For example, populations around the world that have the highest intake of boron have the lowest incidence of arthritis, and boron increases life span in animal studies.

Benefits of Boron

Research indicates that boron works with magnesium and calcium to maintain bone health, increase bone strength and growth, and improve calcium absorption, especially in postmenopausal women. Boron balances vitamin D deficiency (reduces its negative impact) and has a role in cartilage development, which may help prevent arthritis. Supplementation with boron may also have a positive effect on thyroid hormone levels, improve cognitive functioning, and help prevent atherosclerosis.

How to Take Boron Supplements

The Institute of Medicine has not established a daily requirement for boron, but some experts believe 1 mg is the minimum needed for a healthy adult. Doses two to six times that level have been used safely in many studies. Doses of 10 mg or greater can cause nausea, vomiting, rash, diarrhea, and headache.

Best Food Sources

The best dietary sources of boron are applesauce, cooked dried beans and peas, dried fruit, dark green leafy vegetables, grape juice, peanut butter, and nuts. You can get your daily "dose" of boron if you eat just 1.5 ounces of raisins or prunes, or 2 ounces of nuts.

Of Special Interest to Women

The U.S. Department of Agriculture conducted a study in 1999 in which they gave 3 mg of boron to postmenopausal women. After eight days, the women showed 40 percent less loss of calcium and 33 percent less loss of magnesium than before boron supplementation. Other research shows that boron is especially important to bone health in people who are deficient in vitamin D, which is common among older adults. These and similar findings in other studies strongly support including boron in your diet and as a supplement.

CALCIUM

Of all the minerals in the human body, calcium is the most abundant. The average adult carries approximately 1,000 grams of calcium: about 98 percent of it is in bone, 1 percent in teeth, and the remaining amount in the blood and other fluids.

Calcium is a main component of bone, so you need to ensure you get enough to keep your bones strong. However, even the small amount in your bloodstream is critical, because it is necessary for life-sustaining tasks; for example, it is essential for your heart to function properly and for nerve conduction, muscle tone, muscle contractions, and blood clotting. If your body does not get enough calcium, it will extract the mineral from your bones and send it to your bloodstream to make sure those processes take place, thus jeopardizing your bone health.

Benefits of Calcium

Taking calcium can help you "bone up," but it also provides other benefits. Several studies show that calcium can help reduce the risk of colon cancer. In one study, adults who took 700 to 800 mg of calcium daily had a 40 to 50 percent reduced risk of developing the disease. Calcium supplements may also reduce high blood pressure. If you take vitamin D along with calcium, you can get relieve from symptoms of premenstrual syndrome.

How to Take Calcium Supplements

The DRI for calcium for adults is 1,000 to 1,200 mg daily (see page 113.) One of the best-absorbed form of calcium is calcium citrate, which is available in both tablets and liquid; calcium carbonate is the most common form and an acceptable alternative. To determine the amount of elemental calcium your body can absorb from a supplement, look for the Percent Daily Value (%DV) on the label. Every 10 percent in the DV column represents 100 mg of elemental calcium. Therefore, if a calcium supplement has 60 percent of the DV, it contains 600 mg of elemental calcium.

Should you take calcium with or separate from magnesium? Studies show that calcium and magnesium compete with each other for absorption in the intestines, so take these two supplements at least two hours apart.

Best Food Sources

Good sources of calcium are not limited to animal products. Along with cheese, milk, and yogurt, calcium is also found in almonds, beans (black, garbanzo, pinto, etc.), broccoli, calcium-fortified orange juice, figs, leafy greens, raisins, rhubarb, salmon, soy, and tofu.

Of Special Interest to Women

Okay, you know you *need* calcium, but what should you know to ensure you get the most out of the calcium you take?

- Hormone replacement therapy may increase absorption of calcium and decrease its excretion in post-menopausal women.

- The absorption of alendronate (Fosamax) may be jeopardized if you are also taking calcium supplements. Talk to your doctor.

- Calcium can reduce the amount of iron that your body absorbs, so take calcium supplements two hours after any iron-rich food or iron supplement.

- Both vitamins C and D enhance calcium absorption. Take a calcium supplement with orange juice to boost the benefits of both calcium and vitamin C.

CHROMIUM

Chromium is an essential trace mineral that was first discovered in 1797. Its main function is to metabolize carbohydrates, which it does by being an essential component of a compound called glucose tolerance factor (GTF). GTF is composed of chromium (which appears to be the most active of the components), nicotinic acid (niacin), and three amino acids that make up glutathione. Without chromium, GTF could not do its critical work, which is to increase the action of insulin and thus help balance blood glucose levels.

Benefits of Chromium

Many experts believe chromium deficiency is widespread in the United States and is the result of food processing, which strips most foods of natural chromium. This deficiency in turn leads to insulin resistance, which some health care professionals believe can be helped by taking chromium. Chromium may also reduce high cholesterol levels and thus reduce the risk for heart disease and stroke.

How to Take Chromium Supplements

The AI (adequate intake) for chromium is 20 to 25 mcg for women and 30 to 35 mcg for men. Health care professionals often suggest 200 to 400 mcg daily as a supplement. When choosing a chromium supplement from the available forms—chromium picolinate, chromium polynicotinate, chromium chloride, and chromium-enriched yeast—the first two get the nod from most experts because they are best absorbed by the body. Chromium polynicotinate is composed of several molecules of vitamin B_3, which helps stabilize sugar, so this form is preferred by people who take it for diabetes.

Best Food Sources

Although chromium is found naturally in many foods, the amount per serving is typically very small. Accurately identifying how much chromium is in certain foods is not possible because the tools to analyze chromium content are not adequately sensitive. However, the following foods are believed to provide a significant amount of chromium: beer, bran cereals, brewer's yeast, eggs, liver, onions, potatoes, tomatoes, whole grains, and wine.

Of Special Interest to Women

• If you are taking chromium as well as calcium carbonate either as a supplement or in an antacid, the calcium will decrease the absorption of chromium.

• Pregnancy and breast-feeding increases a woman's need for chromium. The AI for pregnant women is 30 mcg; for breast-feeding women, 45 mcg.

COPPER

Copper is a trace element whose total presence in the human body adds up to less than the amount in a penny, but its contribution to your health is priceless (see "Benefits of Copper"). Copper can be found in all the body's tissues, but it is most highly concentrated in the liver. It is the third most abundant trace mineral in the body (iron and zinc rank higher). Copper's absorption is tied with that of zinc, and these two minerals work very closely together to prevent damage from free radicals. In fact, the ratio of copper to zinc, rather than the absolute amount of each mineral alone, makes it possible for a special enzyme called superoxide dismutase (SOD) to prevent cell damage.

Benefits of Copper

A tiny bit of copper goes a long way. Without copper, many critical enzymes would not function properly. Copper plays an essential role in the formation of hemoglobin, bone, and red blood cells, and is needed for proper functioning of the thyroid gland. Copper also has a role in the formation of elastin and collagen, which makes it important for wound healing, and it helps your body produce the skin pigment called melanin.

How to Take Copper Supplements

The DRI for copper for adults is 0.9 mg; for pregnant women, 1.0 mg, and for breast-feeding women, 1.3 mg. Most multivitamin/mineral supplements contain copper (or cupric), which may be in the form of copper picolinic acid, copper gluconate (common), copper glycine, cupric sulfate, or copper lysine. The suggested supplement dose is 1.5 to 3 mg.

Best Food Sources

Foods that provide the highest amounts of copper include asparagus, calf's liver, cashews, crimini mushrooms, eggplant, kale, molasses, mustard greens, oysters, sesame seeds, summer squash, and turnip greens.

Of Special Interest to Women

Infrequently, copper toxicity is a concern because of an increased use of copper water pipes, which can leach the mineral into the drinking water supply. High copper levels in the body, especially when zinc levels are low, may contribute to premenstrual syndrome, fatigue, hypertension, muscle and joint pain, depression, headache, insomnia, abdominal pain, nausea and/or vomiting, and senility. Use of oral contraceptives contributes to high copper levels because they increase absorption of copper.

Postpartum depression has also been linked to high copper levels. During pregnancy, copper concentrations naturally double, and it can take up to three months postpartum for copper concentrations to return to normal. These high copper levels are most likely to affect women who have liver disease or other medical conditions in which bile excretion is compromised.

IRON

Iron is one of the most abundant metals in the human body, and it's essential for life. Nearly two-thirds of the iron resides in hemoglobin, the protein in red blood cells that transports oxygen throughout the tissues. The remaining iron can be found in myoglobin, a protein that supplies oxygen to the muscles; in proteins that store iron for future needs; and in enzymes that are involved in biochemical processes.

Dietary iron is available in two forms: heme and non-heme. Heme iron comes from blood and therefore is found in animal foods; nonheme iron is found in plants such as lentils and beans. Nonheme iron is the form that is added to iron-fortified foods, such as cereals. Although heme iron is absorbed better by the body, it is easy to enhance absorption of nonheme iron.

Benefits of Iron

Iron deficiency among women is reported to be as high as 20 percent, with half of pregnant women believed to be iron-deficient. In many cases, iron levels can be improved by eating more iron-rich foods. If dietary iron isn't enough to restore iron levels, supplements can be used. In either case, additional iron can treat fatigue and iron-deficiency anemia, including anemia associated with heavy menstrual bleeding, pregnancy, and gastrointestinal bleeding. Iron is also needed to make brain chemicals called neurotransmitters, including serotonin, dopamine, and norepinephrine.

How to Take Iron Supplements

The DRI for iron in women ages 19 to 50 is 18 mg; for women who are pregnant, 27 mg; and for breast-feeding women, 9 mg. Once women reach age 51 (around menopause), the requirement is 8 mg. Before starting an iron supplement, you should be tested to determine if you are deficient. Supplements are usually indicated when diet alone cannot restore iron levels within an acceptable time.

Iron supplements are available in two forms: ferrous and ferric. Ferrous fumarate, ferrous sulfate, and ferrous gluconate are the best-absorbed. The term "elemental iron" refers to the amount of iron in a supplement that is available for absorption. Ferrous fumarate, for example, contains 33 percent elemental iron; ferrous sulfate, 20 percent; and ferrous gluconate, 12 percent. If your doctor recommends 60 mg of elemental iron twice daily to treat anemia, for example, you could take one 300 mg tablet of ferrous sulfate (20 percent of 300 mg is 60 mg) two times a day.

Therapeutic doses of iron can cause gastrointestinal side effects, including nausea, vomiting, constipation, and stomach pain. To help minimize side effects, you can start with half the recommended dose and gradually increase it, take your supplements with food, and take divided doses.

Best Food Sources

The best sources of heme iron are beef, chicken liver (high), clams, oysters, and turkey. Nonheme sources include beans (good source; includes black, garbanzo, kidney, pinto, etc.), fortified cereals, lentils, oatmeal, raisins, soybeans, spinach, and tofu.

Of Special Interest to Women

Blood loss during menstruation is the number one cause of low iron levels in women. When iron losses are high, it's important to eat foods that boost absorption of non-heme iron. Foods high in vitamin C—for example, citrus, leafy greens, and tomatoes—significantly enhance the absorption of iron. Lentil soup in a tomato base, oatmeal with fruit, or a glass of orange juice with fortified cereal fits the bill.

Pregnancy increases a woman's iron needs by 1.5 times. If iron intake doesn't meet those needs, iron-deficiency anemia can result, which can lead to premature delivery and low birth weight. Therefore adequate iron intake both prior to and during pregnancy is imperative.

MAGNESIUM

Magnesium is the fourth most abundant mineral in the human body and one of the most "in demand" nutrients. In fact, magnesium plays an essential role in more than 300 enzymatic reactions.

About 65 percent of the body's supply of magnesium is in the skeleton, which explains its importance in bone health. Of the remaining amount, about 27 percent resides in muscle, 6 to 7 percent is found in other cells, and less than 1 percent exists outside the cells. Among some of the non-bone-related functions magnesium performs are the metabolism of fats and carbohydrates, synthesis of DNA and proteins, and the transport of calcium, potassium, and other ions across cell membranes, which impact heart rhythm, nerve health, and muscle contractions.

Benefits of Magnesium

Research results support the importance of maintaining healthy levels of magnesium and of supplementing when necessary. Studies suggest, for example, that low magnesium levels increase the risk of abnormal heart rhythms and that magnesium supplements may reduce the risk of stroke and coronary heart disease. Along the same lines, magnesium helps lower the risk of hypertension, according to the results of a four-year study of more than 30,000 adults. People who have type 2 diabetes often have low magnesium levels, and supplements may help them regulate their blood sugar levels. Healthy levels of magnesium may also help prevent common infections, such as bronchitis, flu, and colds.

How to Take Magnesium Supplements

The Institute of Medicine established that nonpregnant women and breast-feeding women 19 years and older need 310 to 320 mg of magnesium daily, while pregnant women require 350 to 360 mg. Magnesium supplements are often paired with calcium: generally, health care professionals recommend taking calcium and magnesium in a 2:1 ratio (for example, 1,000 mg of calcium and 500 mg of magnesium daily). Calcium and magnesium supplements should be taken at least two hours apart. A typical magnesium supplement dose is 300 to 500 mg daily. Taking more than 750 mg of magnesium per day may cause drowsiness and diarrhea.

Best Food Sources

Foods rich in magnesium are also delicious and include almonds, avocados, bananas, brown rice, greens (e.g., collards, kale, mustard greens, spinach, Swiss chard), hazelnuts, lentils, lima beans, oats, peanuts, soybeans, and tofu.

Of Special Interest to Women

Low magnesium levels can cause or contribute to premenstrual syndrome, menstrual cramps, high blood pressure, insomnia, chronic constipation, kidney stones, and arrhythmia. If you have fibromyalgia, magnesium may help relieve stiff muscles and promote relaxation.

Several studies indicate that magnesium may help prevent and/or treat migraine, which affects a disproportionate number of women. In one study, 600 mg of magnesium taken daily for twelve weeks resulted in a 41.6 percent decrease in frequency of migraine attacks, compared with a 15.8 percent decrease in the placebo group. Patients in the magnesium group also experienced attacks that were briefer and less intense.

MANGANESE

The trace mineral manganese was first identified as an essential nutrient in 1931. Most of the manganese in the body is in the bones, with the remainder in the adrenal glands, kidneys, liver, pancreas, and pituitary gland. Although the human body contains only 15 to 20 milligrams of manganese, the mineral is involved in some important biochemical processes.

Benefits of Manganese

For example, manganese allows the body to use vitamin C, thiamin, biotin, and choline, and it is a catalyst in the production of cholesterol and fatty acids. Manganese is necessary for carbohydrate and protein metabolism, and it activates the enzymes that are involved in bone building. Experts also believe manganese is critical in brain functioning and the production of the thyroid hormone thyroxine.

The enzyme superoxide dismutase (SOD), a potent antioxidant that prevents inflammation and other cell damage from free radicals, cannot function properly without sufficient manganese. Therefore supplements of manganese may boost the work of this critical enzyme. Although evidence is still preliminary, manganese may also help prevent and/or treat allergies, asthma, diabetes, heart disease, osteoporosis, premenstrual syndrome, and rheumatoid arthritis.

How to Take Manganese Supplements

The established Adequate Intake (AI) for manganese is 1.8 mg for women and 2.3 mg for men. The requirement increases to 2.0 mg for pregnant women and 2.6 mg for women who are breast-feeding. Manganese is typically included in multivitamin/mineral and multimineral supplements, although the mineral is also available as a single supplement. Manganese may be in the form of manganese sulfate, chloride, picolinate, gluconate, or amino acid chelate. So far, studies have not shown any one form to be significantly superior.

Best Food Sources

You are sure to find some favorites in this list of best food sources of manganese: brown rice, garlic, garbanzo beans, greens (e.g., chard, kale, mustard greens, spinach), molasses, oats, pineapple, romaine lettuce, raspberries, rye, soybeans, spelt, strawberries, summer squash, tempeh, and turmeric.

Of Special Interest to Women

Women should know a few things about manganese.

- Oral contraceptives and antacids (including those that contain calcium) may interfere with absorption of manganese.

- Manganese has a role in maintaining reproductive health and in the production of breast milk and sex hormones. Therefore, make sure your multivitamin/mineral supplement contains manganese, especially if you are breast-feeding.

- At least one study found that women who consumed levels of manganese below the DRI experienced premenstrual cramping and greater mood swings than women who ate normal or greater amounts of manganese.

PHOSPHORUS

All organisms need phosphorus to perform the basic functions of life. Phosphorus is an essential mineral that is usually found in nature combined with oxygen as phosphate. Living cells use phosphate to transport energy in the body via a compound called adenosine triphosphate, or ATP, which is *the* energy currency of life. Without ATP, your body could not function.

Phosphorus is the second most abundant mineral in the body. Approximately 85 percent of it is found in the bones and teeth, and about 10 percent is in the blood. Although it is efficient on its own, it is more effective when it is joined by vitamins A and D, calcium, iron, and manganese.

Benefits of Phosphorus

In addition to its critical role in energy production, phosphorus also helps the body use carbohydrates, fats, and proteins. Phosphorus is necessary for the growth, maintenance, and repair of cells and for proper kidney function. Signal transmission between nerves depends on phosphorus, as do proper skeletal growth and tooth development.

How to Take Phosphorus Supplements

Because phosphorus is readily available in a great number of common foods, the vast majority of people do not need to take phosphorus supplements. If, however, you have kidney disease or osteomalacia, your health care provider may prescribe a supplement. Some athletes take phosphorus supplements before a strenuous workout or a competition to help reduce fatigue and muscle pain, but this needs to be done with caution (see "Of Special Interest to Women").

Best Food Sources

Foods high in protein are the best sources of phosphorus: beef liver, bran cereals, brewer's yeast, cheese, dried beans (black, garbanzo, kidney, lentils, lima, pinto), milk, nuts, oysters, sardines, whole-grain products, yogurt.

Of Special Interest to Women

When you hear phosphorus, think bone: Phosphorus combines with calcium to help create the foundation of strong bones and teeth. Nutritionists recommend that you balance the calcium and phosphorus in your diet, yet the typical American diet is low in calcium and high in phosphorus. Meat and poultry, for example, contain 10 to 20 times as much phosphorus as calcium, and one serving of a cola beverage can contain 500 mg of phosphorus. If you consume too much phosphorus, your body will excrete the excess and eliminate some calcium along with it.

Although a phosphorus deficiency is rare, women who go on fad or restrictive diets sometimes become deficient. If this sounds like you, your best bet is to switch to a sensible eating plan and include a high-potency multivitamin/mineral that contains phosphorus as part of your lifestyle.

POTASSIUM

Potassium is an electrolyte (a mineral that carries an electric charge and that affects the amount of water in your body, muscle action, and other processes) that works closely with two other electrolytes, sodium and chloride. Unlike sodium and chloride, which are found primarily outside of cells, about 95 percent of the body's potassium resides within the cells. Potassium is very active, however; it must move in and out of cells to conduct its activities. If you have a potassium deficiency or the flow in and out of your cells is blocked, muscle and nerve activity can be seriously compromised.

Benefits of Potassium

Proper muscle and nerve functioning depend on having the right amount of potassium in the body. Potassium regulates how much and how often muscles contract, and it works with sodium to transmit signals in the nervous system. Potassium is necessary to regulate blood pressure and to maintain the body's proper electrolyte balance. Adequate potassium levels are also needed to efficiently store carbohydrates that are used by muscles as fuel.

How to Take Potassium Supplements

The AI for men and women is 4,700 mg, including pregnant women. Breast-feeding women should get 5,100 mg daily. According to the Institute of Medicine, most American women ages 19 to 50 get only about half of the recommended amount of potassium.

Most people can get an adequate amount of potassium from their diet and from their multivitamin/mineral supplement. Your doctor may prescribe a potassium supplement if you are taking a diuretic that is not potassium-sparing, such as Lasix. However, do not ever take potassium supplements without a doctor's supervision. Potassium supplements are available over the counter in a dose of 99 mg. Higher doses can not only irritate your stomach but also upset your electrolyte balance and slow your heart to dangerous levels.

Best Food Sources

Bananas are often the first food that comes to mind when people are asked to name a high-potassium food, yet crimini mushrooms, spinach, Swiss chard, and winter squash pack more potassium per serving than the yellow fruit. Other great sources of potassium include broccoli, brussels sprouts, cantaloupe, fennel, kale, mustard greens, and tomatoes. Avocados, cabbage, cauliflower, halibut, parsley, strawberries, and tuna contain a fair amount of the mineral as well.

Of Special Interest to Women

• Potassium plays a role in bone health because it may counteract the increase in calcium lost in urine caused by a high-salt diet, which many Americans consume.

• Potassium imbalance is a frequent complication of those who go on fad diets (e.g., high-protein diets, liquid diets, single-food diets) and/or lose fluids through excessive exercise or use of saunas, and serious health consequences can result. Signs and symptoms of a potassium deficiency include fatigue, mood swings, muscle weakness, and irregular heartbeat.

SELENIUM

Selenium is an essential trace mineral that is a component of a critically important enzyme called glutathione peroxidase, which is a very potent antioxidant. This mineral is also necessary for normal functioning of the thyroid gland and the immune system. The major dietary source of selenium is plant foods, which get their selenium from the soil. Because selenium levels in soil can vary significantly from region to region, apples grown in upper New York state can have different selenium levels than those grown in Washington state.

Benefits of Selenium

Selenium serves a protective role in the body, shielding red blood cells from free-radical damage, helping produce prostaglandins that reduce inflammation and blood pressure, and fighting the impact of toxic minerals. Studies show that taking supplemental selenium can improve the body's ability to resist viral and bacterial infections. People with

HIV who took 200 mcg of selenium daily for up to two years, for example, had an improvement in symptoms, CD4 T-cell counts, and progression of the virus.

Selenium supplementation may reduce the risk of certain types of cancer, including liver and lung cancer. Some evidence also suggests that selenium may reduce inflammation in the lungs of people with asthma.

How to Take Selenium Supplements

Selenium supplements, whether purchased alone or in a combination product, are available as selenomethionine (best absorbed form), sodium selenite, and sodium selenate. The DRI for selenium for adults is 55 mcg, and the recommended supplement dose is usually 100 to 200 mcg. Chronic low levels of selenium may cause muscle pain, heart disease, and premature aging.

Best Food Sources

Organic foods are much more likely to contain good levels of selenium, so choose organics when possible. The best food sources of selenium are Brazil nuts, brown rice, oats, organ meats, salmon, snapper, sunflower seeds, tuna, and walnuts.

Of Special Interest to Women

- The combination of selenium and vitamins C and E is more effective at preserving bone and preventing osteoporosis than the two vitamins alone, according to a study published in *Clinical Rheumatology*.

- More than 20 percent of menopausal women in the United States have a diagnosed thyroid dysfunction, and millions more are believed to have undiagnosed thyroid problems. Selenium deficiency is a major factor

in low thyroid function, which means you should make
sure you include selenium-rich foods in your diet and
take supplements, if needed.

SULFUR

Sulfur has gotten a bad rap: It's the element in onions
that causes you to tear up when you peel them, and it's
the source of the "aroma" that rises when you cook cabbage and cauliflower. This acid-forming, nonmetallic
element is necessary for human health, even though it
does not hold the title of "essential" mineral. It has not
been assigned a standard DRI value because no specific
deficiency symptoms have been identified. However, it is
an important player in many critical processes in the
body.

Benefits of Sulfur

Sulfur's role in the body is diverse: It helps eliminate toxic
substances, assists the immune system, is key in the synthesis of collagen, and is an important component in hair,
nails, and skin, as well as several amino acids. Many people turn to sulfur supplements to prevent and treat arthritis,
gastrointestinal problems (e.g., diarrhea, constipation, indigestion), seasonal allergies, acne, dry skin, eczema, hemorrhoids, brittle nails, and premenstrual syndrome. Some
of these uses are based on the results of scientific studies,
while others rely on an increasing number of anecdotal accounts.

How to Take Sulfur Supplements

Although no DRI has been established for sulfur, health
care experts have identified beneficial dosages of natural
sulfur supplements in the form of methylsulfonylmethane,
or MSM. This supplement is available as a powder (to be
mixed in liquids), tablets, capsules, and a gel or cream for
topical use.

MSM usually works best when it is taken several times a day with meals, and noticeable results are usually experienced within two to twenty-one days. The suggested individual starting dose is 250 to 500 mg twice a day. You can increase the amount gradually by about 500 mg every three to five days, until you reach a level that brings results. It is not unusual to take 3,000 to 5,000 mg daily and then to gradually reduce the dose once symptoms have been eliminated. When treating arthritis, for example, the suggested dose is up to 5,000 mg daily, which can be enhanced with 250 to 500 mg of vitamin C. MSM has not been found to cause any significant side effects, even at extremely high doses, although some people do report flatulence, heartburn, or a slight feeling of fullness, all of which may be relieved if you take MSM with food.

Best Food Sources

The richest sources of dietary sulfur are egg yolks, garlic, and onions. Other good sources include cabbage, dairy products, fish, legumes, meats, nuts, and wheat germ.

Of Special Interest to Women

Although clinical evidence is sparse, there are many anecdotal reports of how MSM has relieved symptoms of conditions of special concern to women, including fibromyalgia, premenstrual syndrome, irritable bowel syndrome, carpal tunnel syndrome, migraine, and arthritis. These conditions all share a common characteristic, inflammation, which MSM can relieve. MSM also protects and maintains skin, hair, and nail health because sulfur helps the body form the protein keratin, the major component in hair and nails.

ZINC
Zinc is a trace mineral that is needed in small but crucial amounts in the human body. More than half of the body's

supply of zinc is in the muscles; the rest resides mainly in the skin, eyes, bones, prostate, testes, and kidneys.

Zinc plays a key role in growth and sexual maturation. Other important functions include balancing carbohydrate metabolism and blood sugar levels and regulating genetic activity, which it does by "reading" the instructions encoded in the cells' genes. This process is called gene transcription.

Benefits of Zinc

Zinc stimulates the activity of more than a hundred enzymes, including those involved in bone development, thyroid function, tissue growth and repair, protein synthesis, and blood clotting. When cold and flu season approaches, taking zinc can boost the immune system and may reduce the symptoms of the common cold and flu. Many people turn to this antioxidant because it helps protect the macula, the part of the eye that is damaged in macular degeneration.

Research shows zinc supplementation can be helpful in the treatment of anorexia nervosa, which affects a disproportionate number of adolescent girls and women. Other studies have indicated that zinc supplements may benefit chronic hepatitis C, diarrhea, pneumonia, and acute lower respiratory infections.

How to Take Zinc Supplements

The DRIs for zinc are 8 mg for women, 11 mg for pregnant women, and 12 mg for those who are breast-feeding. The most readily absorbed forms of zinc are zinc picolinate, zinc citrate, zinc acetate, and zinc glycerate. Zinc sulfate is the least easily absorbed and can cause stomach upset. Some people who use zinc lozenges to prevent and treat colds report experiencing nausea, stomach pain, mouth irritation, and a bad taste in the mouth.

If you take 40 mg or more of zinc, you may impair iron

and copper absorption. Check the amount of zinc in any supplements you are taking, including multivitamin/minerals. Do not take zinc supplements at the same time you take copper, iron, or phosphorus: separate your zinc dose by two hours from your other supplements.

Best Food Sources

Your best dietary sources of zinc are almonds, calf's liver, dried beans, fortified cereals, milk, oatmeal, oysters, peas, pumpkin seeds, sesame seeds, walnuts, and yogurt.

Of Special Interest to Women

• Zinc supports normal growth and development of the fetus during pregnancy.

• Use of oral contraceptives can reduce your body's ability to absorb zinc.

• If you take high amounts of zinc and do not consume foods high in calcium, the zinc can decrease the amount of calcium you absorb from the intestines into your body.

HERBAL REMEDIES

ALOE VERA

Aloe vera, once known as the "plant of immortality," has been valued for its medicinal benefits since the days of the pharoahs. There are more than 250 varieties of the succulent aloe plant, and most of them are native to northern Africa. The aloe vera (*Aloe barbadensis*) is the variety typically used for its healing properties.

Two parts of the aloe plant are used medicinally: the transparent gel found in the leaves and the latex from the inner lining of the leaves. Each form of aloe has undergone scientific testing and each provides different benefits.

Benefits of Aloe Vera

Enter the kitchen in some homes and you will see an aloe vera plant on the windowsill. That's because the mucilaginous, slightly sticky gel from the leaves is an effective treatment for burns, skin infections, wounds, and other minor skin problems. If you experience a minor cut or burn, a small clipping from an aloe leaf can provide fast relief. In fact, aloe gel has been used for these purposes for thousands of years. Preliminary research in people and animals suggests that topical aloe gel may enhance wound healing and ease inflammation.

An oral form of aloe comes from the dried latex derived from the inner lining of the leaves. The latex contains substances called anthroquinones and anthrones that act like a laxative by increasing movement of stool and the amount of water in the intestines.

How to Use Aloe Vera

Pure aloe vera gel can be applied freely to the skin largely without fear of side effects, and the stickiness of the gel fades quickly. The gel is also available in commercial formulas with other ingredients; however, these products may cause allergic reactions depending on which substances have been added. Oral aloe formulas often contain 10 to 30 mg of hydroxyanthracene derivatives per daily dose, calculated as anhydrous aloin.

The only FDA-approved use of oral aloe vera is as an ingredient in over-the-counter laxatives. The recommended dose is 0.04 to 0.17 g of dried latex. Do not take oral aloe vera for more than seven days, as it may cause diarrhea or worsening of constipation.

ARNICA

Arnica (*Arnica montana*) is a perennial herb that is native to the mountains of Europe and Siberia and now also grows in the northern United States and Canada. Its yellow-orange daisylike flowers have been used for healing purposes since the 1500s, when it was popular among the Native Americans and Europeans as a treatment for muscle pain, inflammation, and wounds.

Benefits of Arnica

Today arnica is used primarily as a topical remedy to reduce the swelling and pain associated with trauma (including after surgery), sprains, bruises, and muscle and joint problems, including arthritis, carpal tunnel syndrome, and fibromyalgia. Organic chemicals called sesquiterpene lactones and flavonoid glycosides are believed to be responsible for arnica's ability to reduce inflammation and pain.

How to Use Arnica

Arnica is available as a topical cream and ointment in strengths of 20 to 25 percent tincture. It can be applied once daily but should not be used on skin abrasions or open wounds. Side effects may include redness or irritation where the cream is applied. Long-term use may cause eczema, peeling, or blisters. Anyone who is allergic to sunflowers, marigolds, or chamomile may be allergic to arnica.

Of Special Interest to Women

Arnica use cannot be recommended during pregnancy or breast-feeding because of the lack of scientific evidence.

ASTRAGALUS

Astragalus (*Astragalus membranaceus*) is a popular herb in traditional Chinese medicine, where it has been used for thousands of years to protect the body against infection and disease. This perennial plant is a native of northern and eastern China, as well as Korea and Mongolia. The roots are the healing portion of the plant.

Benefits of Astragalus

Recent research has found that astragalus has diuretic, anti-inflammatory, and antibacterial abilities. The antioxidants in astragalus support the immune system and suggest the herb may help prevent colds, flu, and respiratory infections. Studies in China indicate that the herb may relieve symptoms of heart disease, improve heart function, and reduce blood glucose levels in people who have type 2 diabetes. There are also indications that it may help fight cancer.

How to Use Astragalus

Astragalus supplements are available as capsules (which contain the powdered extract), tincture, ointment, fluid extract, and as dried root for tea. Suggested doses are as follows:

- Tea: 3 to 6 g of dried root steeped in 12 ounces of water, drunk up to three times a day

- Tincture: 1:5 solution in 30 percent ethanol, 3 to 5 mL taken three times daily

- Powdered root: 500 to 1,000 mg three to four times daily

- Fluid extract: 1:1 solution in 25 percent ethanol, 2 to 4 mL taken three times daily

Astragalus may interact with certain medications. Talk to your doctor before using astragalus if you are taking any of the following:

- *Anticoagulants.* Astragalus may increase the effects of these drugs and increase your risk of bleeding.

- *Antiviral drugs.* Astragalus may increase the effects

of these medications, such as acyclovir and inter-
feron.

- *Diabetes medications.* Astragalus may lower blood
  sugar levels, which will make the drug effect stronger.

- *Diuretics.* Astragalus may increase the impact of other
  diuretics.

- *High blood pressure medications.* Astragalus may reduce blood pressure, which in turn may increase the
  effect of these drugs.

BLACK COHOSH

Native American women of centuries past dealt with the
symptoms of their menstrual cycles and other gynecological conditions by using an herb called black cohosh
(*Actaea racemosa,* formerly *Cimicifuga racemosa*), and
women today are doing the same. The roots and rhizomes
of black cohosh contain terpene glycoside, which appears
to be the active factor in this native herb of North America.

Benefits of Black Cohosh

The American College of Obstetrics and Gynecology supports the use of black cohosh for relief of menopausal
symptoms, especially for mood swings, sleep disturbances,
and hot flashes. Many women also use black cohosh to relieve similar symptoms associated with premenstrual syndrome, including headache, night sweats, cramping, and
bloating.

How to Use Black Cohosh

Supplements of black cohosh should be standardized to
contain 1 mg of terpene glylcosides per 20 mg tablet.
Most studies of black cohosh have used a daily dose of
40 mg or 80 mg with similar results using both dosages.

Black cohosh is available in tablets and as a tincture. The British Herbal Compendium recommends 0.4 to 2 mL of a 60 percent alcohol tincture daily. It usually takes four to eight weeks to experience the full benefits of black cohosh.

Infrequently black cohosh may cause side effects, including constipation, low blood pressure, nausea, and vomiting. High doses of black cohosh may cause dizziness, headache, or visual problems. Consult your doctor before using black cohosh if you have high blood pressure, a seizure disorder, a history of blood clots or stroke, liver disease, or an allergy to aspirin.

Of Special Interest to Women

- Because black cohosh has not been adequately tested during pregnancy, you should not use this herb while pregnant unless you have talked to your health care provider.

- The American College of Obstetricians and Gynecologists states that black cohosh may be helpful in the short term (six months or less) for relief of menopausal symptoms. No longer-term studies have yet been conducted.

- Although it is still unclear if black cohosh is safe for women who have hormone-related disease such as breast cancer, recent research indicates that it has beneficial effects similar to those of SERMs—selective estrogen receptor modulators.

BOSWELLIA

The Ayurvedic herb boswellia (*Boswellia serrata*), also known as Indian frankincense, comes from the boswellia tree, which is a native of India. Scientific research has identified several components of boswellia that seem to be responsible for its anti-inflammatory and antiarthritic qualities: boswellic acid and alpha-boswellic acid. These ingredients are found in the gummy resin that is derived from the tree.

Benefits of Boswellia

Recent studies have found that boswellia can be effective in the treatment of arthritis, asthma, and ulcerative colitis. Boswellia appears to inhibit inflammation by blocking the synthesis of leukotrienes, substances that cause inflammation by promoting free-radical damage and other harmful activities.

How to Use Boswellia

Boswellia is available as tablets and capsules. Look for a standardized extract of boswellic acids of at least 37.5 percent. A typical dose for arthritis is 400 mg of an extract with 37.5 percent boswellic acids, taken three times daily.

Rare side effects include diarrhea, rash, and nausea. No drug interactions are known at this time.

Of Special Interest to Women

If you are pregnant or breast-feeding, talk to your doctor before using boswellia.

BROMELAIN

Bromelain is a substance derived from the fruit and stem of pineapples. It contains enzymes that help digest proteins as well as enzymes that block the production of substances called kinins that form during inflammation.

Benefits of Bromelain

Bromelain can provide two general types of relief, depending on when you take it. If you take bromelain with meals, it assists in the digestion of proteins and can help relieve gastrointestinal symptoms, including heartburn and symptoms of irritable bowel syndrome. If you take it on an empty stomach, it acts as an anti-inflammatory and can reduce swelling and the pain that often accompanies it, as in arthritis, bursitis, and fibromyalgia.

How to Use Bromelain

Various doses are recommended depending on the condition being treated. A typical dose for adults is from 250 to 750 mg three times a day. For joint inflammation, many health care professionals recommend 500 to 2,000 mg per day in divided doses. As a digestive aid, a typical dose is 500 mg in divided doses taken with meals.

Bromelain supplements are available as tablets, capsules, and powder. Their activity is measured in GDUs (gelatin digesting units) or MCUs (milk clotting units). Look for products that contain 4 GDUs or 6 MCUs per milligram.

Do not take bromelain if you are allergic to pineapple, if you are taking antibiotics, or if you have high blood pressure or liver or kidney disease. Do not use bromelain for more than eight to ten consecutive days.

Of Special Interest to Women

Do not use bromelain if you are pregnant or breast-feeding. Although allergic reactions to bromelain are very rare, some of the symptoms of such reactions include heavy menstrual bleeding and nonmenstrual bleeding from the uterus.

BUTTERBUR

The butterbur plant (*Petasites hybridus*) is a perennial found throughout Europe, Asia, and North America. Extracts of the plant have been used for more than two thousand years to treat pain, fever, and spasms. Its active ingredients are sesquiterpenes, including petasin and isopetasin.

Benefits of Butterbur

Today butterbur is used primarily for migraine, asthma, and incontinence. For example, several double-blind, placebo-controlled trials totaling more than 300 patients have shown butterbur to significantly reduce migraine attacks: More than 66 percent of all patients had a 50 percent or greater reduction in episodes.

How to Use Butterbur

When buying a butterbur supplement, make sure it is free of pyrrolizidine alkaloids (PAs), a naturally occurring ingredient that can cause liver damage. Manufacturers typically process PAs out of their products. The extract is usually standardized to contain a minimum of 7.5 mg of petasin and isopetasin. The typical adult dose is 50 to 100 mg twice daily with meals.

Butterbur may prevent migraine, not treat it. It typically takes about two months of daily use before noting results. Side effects are rare; if they occur, they are usually mild and may include headache, drowsiness, nausea, vomiting, itchy eyes, fatigue, and diarrhea.

Of Special Interest to Women

If you are pregnant or breast-feeding, talk to your doctor before using butterbur.

CALENDULA

Calendula (*Calendula officinalis*), better known as marigold, is a flowering plant that has been used for medicinal purposes since the twelfth century or earlier. This annual plant grows best in Europe, Western Asia, and the

United States. Its relatives include ragweed, daisies, and chrysanthemums. The dried petals of its orange-yellow flowers have traditionally been used to relieve symptoms of ulcers, stomach upset, and menstrual cramps.

Benefits of Calendula

Calendula contains high levels of antioxidants called flavonoids, which can protect the body against cell damage. Experts are not certain if these substances or others give this plant its antibacterial, anti-inflammatory, and antiviral properties. However, today calendula is used mainly to treat acne, hemorrhoids, burns, cuts, bruises, and minor infections. Studies suggest that calendula is effective because it increases blood flow to the treated areas and it helps produce collagen proteins, which assist in healing the skin.

How to Use Calendula

Calendula ointment, available in strengths ranging from 2 to 10 percent tincture of calendula, can be applied to affected skin three to four times daily, as needed. Do not apply it to open wounds. If you are allergic to daisies, ragweed, or chrysanthemums, you may have an allergic reaction (rash) to calendula.

Of Special Interest to Women

You should not use calendula if you are pregnant or breast-feeding because this herb can affect the menstrual cycle. Theoretically this herb may also have a negative impact on conception.

CAPSAICIN

Chili peppers (cayenne peppers) are the source of capsaicin, an alkaloid that is known for its fiery effect when it makes contact with the skin or the mucus membranes of the body. Capsaicin works by decreasing the amount of substance P, a neurotransmitter that passes along pain signals from the skin to the brain.

Benefits of Capsaicin

Capsaicin can be used to treat minor muscle and joint pain as well as nerve pain. Thus it can relieve the pain of arthritis, backache, diabetic neuropathy, neuralgia, shingles, and sprains. It also has been used to reduce postsurgical pain in cancer patients.

How to Use Capsaicin

Capsaicin is available as a gel, lotion, cream, liquid, and pads that can be applied to the skin. It can be purchased in a range of strengths from 0.025 percent to 0.075 percent. Typically, apply capsaicin three to four times daily. Always wear gloves when using capsaicin and wash your hands with soap and water after applying it to avoid getting the substance into your eyes or other sensitive body parts.

When you use capsaicin, you will likely feel a stinging, burning, or warm sensation on the treated area. This is a normal reaction and usually subsides and disappears after the first few days of treatment, but it may last longer. You must use capsaicin every day to reap its benefits. It may take several weeks before you experience significant relief, although you can expect some reduction in symptoms before that time. Never use on broken skin.

CHAMOMILE

Two types of chamomile are used for their healing powers: German and Roman. Because the German variety is used more often in the United States, we focus on this variety. German chamomile (*Matricaria recutita*) is a member of the daisy family, and its flowers are used to make the herbal supplements.

Benefits of Chamomile

Traditionally chamomile has been used to treat mouth ulcers, skin irritation, and general anxiety, and it is still used for these purposes today. Recently it has shown some promise in the fight against cancer. Chamomile is often the sole ingredient or one of the ingredients in teas recommended to help people who have trouble falling or staying asleep.

How to Use Chamomile

Chamomile is available as a tea and as capsules, tablets, liquid extract, and tincture. Common dosages are as follows:

- Tea: 1 to 4 cups daily from tea bags

- Capsules/tablets: 400 to 1,600 mg daily, taken in divided doses

- Liquid extract: 1:1 in 45 percent alcohol, 1 to 4 mL taken three times daily

- Tincture: 1:5 in alcohol, 15 mL taken three to four times daily

Side effects of chamomile use may include rash or shortness of breath. You should not use chamomile if you have an allergy to other plants in the Asteraceae family (e.g., aster, mums, mugwort, ragweed).

Of Special Interest to Women

In theory, chamomile may stimulate the uterus, so it should not be used during pregnancy. Because no studies have been done on its impact during breast-feeding, you should not use this herb if you are nursing.

CHASTE TREE BERRY

Chaste tree berry (*Vitex agnus-castus*), also known as vitex, is the fruit of the chaste tree, a small shrublike tree that grows in Central Asia and the Mediterranean area. The story goes that monks in the Middle Ages used chaste tree berry to reduce sexual desire, hence the name of the plant.

Benefits of Chaste Tree Berry

Today it is women, not men, who use chaste tree berry. The herb provides relief from symptoms associated with premenstrual syndrome, menopause, acne, fibrocystic breast, and endometriosis. It is also helpful in some cases of infertility.

How to Use Chaste Tree Berry

The dried ripe berries of the plant are used to prepare tablets, capsules, and tinctures. The typical dose is three cups of tea daily (made by pouring 8 ounces of boiling water onto 1 teaspoon of ripe berries and steeping for 10 minutes). If you use the tincture, take 1 mL three times daily.

Chaste tree berry may cause mild side effects, including rash, dizziness, or gastrointestinal discomfort.

Of Special Interest to Women

Chaste tree berry may affect hormone levels. Therefore, if you are pregnant, taking birth control pills, or have a hormone-related condition (e.g., breast cancer), do not use this herb.

CINNAMON

The cinnamon in your Danish or on your applesauce not only tastes good, it has healing qualities as well. Cinnamon comes from the bark of the tropical evergreen cinnamon tree and contains three main components in its essential oils. These substances are believed to be responsible for this spice's ability to improve health.

Benefits of Cinnamon

Cinnamon may help reduce inflammation, stop bacterial growth, lower cholesterol and triglyceride levels, prevent clumping of blood platelets, and improve the body's response to insulin in type 2 diabetes. Some preliminary studies suggest cinnamon may also help improve cognitive functioning.

In a study published in *Diabetes Care,* sixty adults with type 2 diabetes were given 1, 3, or 6 grams of cinnamon daily or a placebo for 40 days. The people who took cinnamon had an 18 to 29 percent reduction in their glucose (sugar) levels, as well as reduced cholesterol and triglyceride levels.

How to Use Cinnamon

Cinnamon is easy to use: Just add ground cinnamon to your favorite foods. As little as 1/2 teaspoon (about 1 gram) daily may reduce blood sugar levels by 20 to 25 percent. If you prefer to use a cinnamon tincture, use 2 to 3 mL three times daily. For capsules, use the equivalent of 3 to 6 grams of ground cinnamon daily.

In rare cases, cinnamon may cause bronchial constriction or rash. Cinnamon is not known to interact with medications.

Of Special Interest to Women

If you are pregnant, you should avoid use of cinnamon oil or high doses of cinnamon bark, as it may induce miscarriage.

CURCUMIN
Curcumin is one of the main active phytonutrients in turmeric, a spice that is derived from the rhizomes of *Cur-*

cuma longa, a member of the ginger family. Turmeric has been used both as a traditional Indian and Chinese medicine since the seventh century A.D., when it was valued for treating inflammatory conditions such as arthritis, as well as diarrhea, fever, colds, leprosy, and bladder and kidney inflammation. The old custom of making turmeric paste and applying it to the skin is now being investigated as a way to prevent skin cancer.

Benefits of Curcumin

Researchers have found that the ancient uses for curcumin were on target, at least when it comes to inflammatory conditions such as arthritis. Although only a few human studies have been done, hundreds of other experiments have shown that curcumin has the ability to stop or prevent certain types of cancer, reduce inflammation, improve cardiovascular health, prevent gallstones, and kill or inhibit certain disease-causing organisms. Recently curcumin has been found to normalize blood sugar levels and restore enzymes that are involved in blood sugar metabolism. Some preliminary research indicates that curcumin may have a role in the prevention of Alzheimer's disease as well.

How to Use Curcumin

Will the curry powder in your spice rack provide you with enough curcumin? Although curry powder contains turmeric, the amount of curcumin is variable and usually very low. To ensure results, shop for curcumin supplements that are standardized to contain 95% curcuminoids. A typical dose is 200 to 400 mg taken three times daily for inflammatory conditions. You can enhance the absorption of curcumin if you take an equal amount of bromelain. If you use tea, 1 to 1.5 g of dried turmeric root may be steeped in 8 ounces of water for 15 minutes and used twice daily.

Curcumin may cause stomach upset, especially if used in high doses or taken for a prolonged time.

Of Special Interest to Women

The safety of curcumin in pregnant and breast-feeding women has not been determined.

DANDELION

Dandelion (*Taraxacum officinale*) is a perennial herb with long, toothed leaves, which gave this plant its name ("dent-de-lion" means "lion's tooth" in Old French). The plant grows throughout the temperate parts of Europe, North America, and Asia. In North America, Native Americans used this herb to treat kidney disease and heartburn, while traditional Chinese medicine values it for hepatitis and upper respiratory infections. Although today many people call the dandelion a weed, others realize its medicinal and nutritional benefits.

Benefits of Dandelion

Dandelion leaf is a natural diuretic, and it has an advantage over many other diuretics because the herb is a good source of potassium, a substance that is often depleted from the body when other diuretics are used. Some women with premenstrual syndrome say that dandelion relieves bloating and water retention.

The roots of dandelion are used to stimulate appetite, relieve constipation and flatulence, and enhance digestion. Some health care professionals claim dandelion can detoxify the gallbladder and liver as well as regulate blood sugar levels and cholesterol levels, although more research is needed in these areas.

How to Use Dandelion

Dandelion is available as dried root (for use as tea), leaf fluid extract, root tincture, and capsules containing dried herb. Typical doses are 1,000 to 3,000 mg of dried herb (in capsules) taken in divided doses daily, 4 to 8 mL daily of a

1:1 leaf fluid extract in 25 percent alcohol, or 1 to 2 teaspoons daily of a 1:5 root tincture in 45 percent alcohol.

The most common reported side effects are skin allergy, eczema, or increased sensitivity to the sun. People
who are allergic to chamomile, feverfew, ragweed, sunflowers, daisies, mums, and other members of the Asteraceae family may be allergic to dandelion as well. Do not
take dandelion supplements if you have intestinal or bile
duct blockage or inflammation of the gallbladder.

FEVERFEW

Feverfew (*Tanacetum parthenium*) is an herb that derives
its name from the Latin word "febrifugia," or "fever reducer." This member of the sunflower family is a native of
southeastern Europe, but today it can be found throughout
the continent. It has yellow daisy-like flowers, but the
yellow-green leaves are the most often used for remedies.

Benefits of Feverfew

European folk medicine practitioners valued feverfew for
its ability to treat headache, arthritis, and fever. Today the
emphasis is on its ability to relieve symptoms of migraine
and other headache pain. A compound called parthenolide,
which can calm smooth muscle spasms, appears to be responsible for this relief. Parthenolide also inhibits the activity of substances that cause inflammation. Although studies
using feverfew for arthritis have not been promising, trials
using it for eczema resulted in relief from inflammation.

How to Use Feverfew

Feverfew is available as capsules, tablets, and extracts
made from dried feverfew. You can buy loose dried leaves
to make tea, or find a source of raw, fresh leaves. The dried
extract should be standardized to contain 0.2 to 0.4%
parthenolides. Studies typically use 50 to 100 mg daily to
prevent migraines, and up to 250 mg can be used without

causing side effects. It usually takes four to six weeks of daily use of feverfew before it is effective. To make tea, place 1 teaspoon of dried leaves in 6 ounces of water, boil for 5 to 10 minutes, and strain the leaves from the tea. Drink several cups per day.

Side effects from feverfew may include abdominal pain, diarrhea, indigestion, nausea, vomiting, and nervousness. Chewing the raw leaves may cause mouth ulcers and swelling of the lips, tongue, and mouth. If you are allergic to chamomile, ragweed, or yarrow, you may also be allergic to feverfew.

If you have a bleeding disorder or are taking blood-thinning medications, do not use feverfew without first consulting your doctor. Once you begin taking feverfew, do not stop abruptly if you have used it for more than one week, as you may experience withdrawal symptoms such as rebound headache, fatigue, joint pain, and anxiety.

Of Special Interest to Women

If you are pregnant, do not use feverfew because it may cause uterine contractions and increase the risk of premature delivery or miscarriage.

FLAXSEED

Flaxseed comes from the flax plant (*Linum usitatissimum*), which has populated the planet since the Stone Ages. The seeds are slightly larger than sesame seeds and have a hard, shiny, smooth shell. It seems appropriate that their Latin name means "most useful," as these seeds, especially when ground, have both medicinal and nutritional value. In fact, the ancient Greeks and Romans valued them for their healing powers and culinary uses.

Benefits of Flaxseed

The many benefits offered by flaxseed are largely due to the presence of alpha-linolenic acid (ALA) and lignan, a type of phytoestrogen and antioxidant that also provides fiber. Flaxseed is rich in the omega-3 fatty acid ALA, which is a precursor to the omega-3 found in fish oils called eicosa-pentaenoic acid (EPA). For people who don't want to eat fish or take fish oil supplements, flaxseed is a good alternative.

Research shows that ALA, along with the lignans, either separately or combined, makes flaxseed valuable for its ability to reduce inflammation, lower cholesterol levels, decrease blood pressure, and help prevent or treat a wide variety of conditions, including breast cancer, constipation, endometriosis, dry eyes, gallstones, hemorrhoids, menopause, and osteoporosis, among others.

How to Use Flaxseed

Flaxseed should be ground to maximize its digestability and nutritional value. Buy whole flaxseed and grind it in a coffee grinder at home, or purchase it already ground. Include 1 to 2 tablespoons of ground flaxseed in your diet every day: sprinkle it on cereal, stir it into smoothies, add it to stews and casseroles, include it in homemade muffins and bread, and use it as a topping on steamed vegetables.

Of Special Interest to Women

When the lignans in flaxseed reach the intestinal tract, bacteria convert them into two hormonelike substances called enterolactone and enterodiol. These agents appear to protect against breast cancer, based on results of animal studies and on the fact that a vegetarian diet is associated with a lower risk of breast cancer. Research shows that women with breast cancer and women who eat meat and other animal products typically excrete significantly less lignans than vegetarian women who don't have breast cancer.

GARLIC

Garlic (*Allium sativum*) is one of the most popular and best-selling herbal supplements in the United States. Although it has been valued since ancient times for its healing qualities, Louis Pasteur gave the herb a big boost in 1858 when he discovered its ability to kill disease-causing bacteria.

Researchers believe the substances that give garlic its unique taste and smell are the same ones that provide its health benefits. The substances are called organosulfur compounds, and investigators are exploring how they may be useful in preventing and treating chronic diseases such as cancer and heart disease. But garlic has already proven itself in other areas.

Benefits of Garlic

Study results are not consistent, but in many cases garlic has effectively lowered cholesterol levels, reduced high blood pressure, and destroyed various microorganisms. A 2007 report, for example, found garlic to be effective against *Candida albicans,* which causes vaginal infections. Another 2007 study supported the use of garlic to help lower cholesterol, improve heart function, and prevent blood clots.

How to Use Garlic

Garlic is beneficial both as a food and a supplement. The recommended dose is 4 g (1 to 2 cloves) of raw garlic daily, one 300 mg capsule or tablet of dried garlic powder (standardized to 1.3 percent alliin or 0.6 percent allicin) two to three times daily, or 7.2 g of aged garlic extract daily. Deodorized supplements are available.

No major side effects are associated with normal use of garlic. Some people experience flatulence, bloating, bad breath, diarrhea, nausea, or heartburn when they first use garlic, but these symptoms usually disappear with continued use and/or by reducing the dose.

Garlic reduces the blood's ability to clot, so excessive amounts may cause abnormal bleeding if it is used along with anticoagulant or antiplatelet drugs. It may also interact with herbs that affect blood clotting, such as devil's claw, ginger, gingko, horse chestnut, and red clover.

Of Special Interest to Women

A study conducted in 1995 found that the amniotic fluid samples obtained from pregnant women who had ingested capsules containing garlic oil had a significant odor of garlic. This study is similar to later ones in which researchers investigated the impact of a nursing mother's diet on which fruits and vegetables her infant would accept as part of its diet. Apparently, breast-feeding mothers who eat vegetables are more likely to have children who eat vegetables as well.

GINGER

Ginger (*Zingiber officinale*) is a tropical plant that is one of the most popular herbs in the world today. The plant has green-purple flowers and a fragrant underground stem (rhizome) that is used for both culinary and medicinal purposes. Ginger has been a part of herbal medicine traditions in Asia, India, and Arabic countries since ancient times, where it has been used for stomachache, nausea, diarrhea, arthritis, and heart conditions. The ingredients in ginger that are believed to provide its benefits are volatile oils and phenol compounds, such as gingerols and shogaols.

Benefits of Ginger

Perhaps the most common medicinal use of ginger is to prevent or treat nausea, whether it is caused by pregnancy (morning sickness), chemotherapy, motion, or surgery. The majority of studies in which ginger was used for nausea found it to be effective when compared with placebo and equally or somewhat less effective than antinausea medications, although it did provide good relief. People who want an alternative to medications can turn to ginger. Ginger has also been used for gastrointestinal disorders such as irritable bowel syndrome and for arthritis, menstrual cramps, and general joint and muscle pain.

How to Use Ginger

Ginger is available as fresh or dried root powder, liquid extracts (tinctures), tablets, capsules, and teas. Do not ingest more than 2 to 4 grams of ginger per day (this includes ginger in your food). For nausea and other gastrointestinal problems or arthritis pain, take 2 to 4 g of fresh root daily (0.25 to 1.0 g of powdered root) or 1.5 to 3.0 mL (30 to 90 drops) of tincture daily. To make a tea, steep 2 tablespoons of freshly shredded ginger in boiling water for 5 to 10 minutes; drink two to three times daily. Tea is usually recommended for cold and flu symptoms and menstrual cramps.

Ginger rarely causes side effects when it is used in small doses. Powdered ginger is the form most often associated with side effects, which may include bloating, gas, heartburn, and nausea.

Of Special Interest to Women

If you are pregnant and have morning sickness or hyperemesis gravidarum, you can safely use capsules of ginger root powder for up to five days at a dose of 75 mg to 1 g daily in divided doses. Ginger contains substances that could theoretically cause birth defects if taken in large amounts. No increase in birth defects has been seen in studies that used 1 gram of ginger daily.

GINKGO

Ginkgo (*Ginkgo biloba*) refers to both the herb and the tree from which the herb is derived. The ginkgo tree is the oldest living tree species known, and individual trees have been known to live as long as a thousand years. Its seeds have been used as food and medicine for more than four millennia. Traditional Chinese medicine herbalists still use ginkgo to treat asthma, bronchitis, and brain disorders. Researchers are investigating these and other uses for the herb.

Benefits of Ginkgo

As an antioxidant, ginkgo prevents free-radical damage to cell membranes and helps maintain the integrity of blood vessel walls, which improves blood flow to the brain, limbs, and other areas that are supplied by capillaries. Ginkgo also supports circulation by inhibiting the effects of a blood clotting substance that has been linked to allergies, asthma, inflammatory problems, and cardiovascular diseases. Studies show that standardized ginkgo extract relieves ringing in the ears and enhances brain function.

How to Use Ginkgo

Ginkgo is available as capsules, tea, and tablets. Typical dosage is 80 to 240 mg of a 50:1 standardized leaf extract taken daily in two to three divided doses. Look for products that have been standardized to 24 percent to 25 percent ginkgo flavone glycosides and 6 percent terpine lactones, the herb's active ingredients.

Side effects of ginkgo may include skin reactions, diarrhea, dizziness, headache, gastrointestinal upset, and nausea. Because some data indicate that ginkgo may increase the risk of bleeding, you should not use this herb if you are taking anticoagulant drugs or if you have a bleeding disorder. Talk to your doctor or dentist before undergoing surgery or dental procedures if you are taking ginkgo.

Of Special Interest to Women

Do not use ginkgo if you are pregnant or breast-feeding, as there is no reliable research on its safety. The risk of bleeding associated with ginkgo may pose a danger during pregnancy.

GINSENG

Asian ginseng (*Panax ginseng*), also known as Chinese ginseng or Korean ginseng, has been one of the most commonly used herbs in traditional Chinese medicine and other systems of medicine for many centuries. Note that Asian ginseng and American ginseng (*Panax quinquefolius*) are types of true ginseng, while Siberian ginseng (*Eleutherococcus senticosus*) is not.

Both the Asian and American varieties offer similar benefits, which is fortunate, as Asian ginseng is nearly extinct in nature although it is cultivated, while the American variety is more readily available both in the wild and through cultivation. We use "ginseng" to refer to both types.

Benefits of Ginseng

The root of ginseng contains ginsenosides (or panaxosides), which are believed to possess the herb's medicinal properties. The best studied use of ginseng is for type 2 diabetes (it reduces blood glucose levels) and mental functioning (a modest improvement in thinking and memory). A few studies suggest it may boost the immune system, prevent some types of cancer, reduce fatigue, lower blood pressure, and improve stamina. Siberian ginseng helps the body adapt to stress; it also may enhance physical endurance and mental acuity.

How to Use Ginseng

The dried root of ginseng is used to make capsules, tablets, extracts, and teas. A cream is also available for topical use. Ginseng extracts may be standardized to 4 to 7 percent ginsenosides, although independent testing of ginseng supplements has found that many brands do not contain the claimed level of ginsenosides. Look for reputable brands when purchasing ginseng.

Typical dosages are 100 to 200 mg of a standardized ginseng extract (4 percent ginsenosides) once or twice daily or 0.5 to 2 g of dry ginseng root, taken daily in divided doses. For the fluid extract or tincture, the typical dose is 1 to 2 mL daily of a 1:1 extract or 5 to 10 mL of a 1:5 tincture taken daily. Regardless of which ginseng form you choose, do not take it continuously for more than two to three weeks. After that time, take a break for one to two weeks before starting again.

Most people tolerate ginseng very well. Side effects occur infrequently and may include rash, itching, diarrhea, sore throat, excitability, anxiety, depression, or insomnia. Ginseng may lower blood sugar levels, and this effect may be greater in people who have diabetes than in those who do not. If you have diabetes, be aware of this possibility and adjust your medication if needed if you are not taking ginseng specifically to lower blood sugar levels.

Of Special Interest to Women

- Despite claims that ginseng can increase libido in women, there are no data to back them up.

- Ginseng has a mild estrogenic effect, which means the herb may increase symptoms in women who have estrogen-sensitive problems such as fibrocystic breast changes or uterine fibroids.

• Do not use ginseng if you are pregnant or breast-feeding.

GREEN TEA

Green tea (*Camellia sinesis*) has been enjoyed as a beverage for as many as 500,000 years, according to archeologists. It was first cultivated in China and India, where it was used in traditional Chinese and Indian medicine as a diuretic and to boost energy, improve heart health, heal wounds, enhance the mind, and promote digestion. Today, researchers are discovering a scientific basis for some of these claims, and more.

Black tea is prepared from fully fermented tea leaves, oolong tea is made from partially fermented leaves, and green tea comes from unfermented leaves. Of the three types of tea, green tea contains the highest concentration of potent antioxidants called polyphenols, which are the source of its healing qualities. In contrast, the more tea leaves are fermented, the lower their polyphenol content and the greater their caffeine content.

Benefits of Green Tea

The main polyphenol in green tea is EGCG—epigallocatechin gallate. Studies in both animals and humans show that EGCG and other green tea polyphenols have anti-inflammatory and anticancer properties. Researchers found, for example, that green tea reduces total cholesterol and raises "good" cholesterol, reduces inflammation associated with Crohn's disease and ulcerative colitis, inhibits the growth of breast cancer cells, may prevent the onset and growth of skin tumors, and may prevent obesity and atherosclerosis.

How to Use Green Tea

Green tea can be enjoyed in the traditional way—two to three cups per day (for a total of 240 to 320 mg polyphenols)—or you can take a standardized green tea extract in capsules, 300 to 400 mg daily. Look for supplements that provide the highest percentage of polyphenols per dose, preferably 70 percent or higher of polyphenols.

Of Special Interest to Women

Some women are concerned about drinking green tea during pregnancy because of the caffeine, even though it contains significantly less than do black tea and coffee. Well-known complementary physician and author Andrew Weil, MD, notes that there is no evidence that consuming 200 mg of caffeine per day from green tea or other beverages increases a woman's risk of miscarriage. Brewed green tea typically contains 30 to 50 mg of caffeine per 8-ounce serving.

Another concern about green tea and pregnancy is that EGCG may impact how the body uses folate, which is critical in preventing birth defects in babies. The problem is that EGCG molecules are similar in structure to methotrexate, a substance that kills cancer cells by attaching itself to an enzyme called dihydrofolate reductase (DHFR). The EGCG in green tea also binds with DHFR, which shuts down the enzyme and thus reduces the body's ability to use folate optimally. No one knows how much green tea you have to drink before it makes an impact on folate. Thus some women choose to limit green tea consumption to one or two cups daily or they eliminate it altogether until they give birth.

HAWTHORN

Hawthorn (*Crataegus oxycantha;* also known as *C. laevigata*) has been popular since ancient times as an herb that benefits the heart. The word "hawthorn" refers to a large genus of shrubs and trees that is native to northern Europe, Asia, and North America. There are dozens of hawthorn species, but *C. oxycantha* is the one most often used in Western medicine. The berries, leaves, and flowers are used to make extracts for supplements.

Benefits of Hawthorn

It appears our ancient ancestors were right in their claim that hawthorn is good for the heart, although they didn't have a scientific explanation for it. We now know why: Hawthorn has bioflavonoids such as quercetin, hyperoside, and oligomeric procyanidins. The procyanidins, for example, help relax the blood vessels, which enhances blood flow. Hawthorn has been used successfully to treat heart failure, to reduce symptoms of coronary artery disease (e.g., angina), to help maintain blood pressure, and for kidney and digestive problems.

Hawthorn works gradually; you can expect it to take several months of daily use before you reap this herb's benefits.

How to Use Hawthorn

Hawthorn is available as liquid extract, capsules, tablets, and crushed leaves or fruits for infusions. Look for extracts standardized for total bioflavonoid content (usually 2.2 percent) or procyanidins (usually 18.75 percent). Dosages range from 80 to 300 mg of the extract in capsules or tablets taken two to three times daily, or 4 to 5 mL of tincture taken three times daily. The tincture is bitter, so add honey or lemon to mask the taste. To make an infusion, use 2 teaspoons of crushed leaves or fruits per 8 ounces of boiling water. Steep for 20 minutes and drink two cups daily.

Hawthorn is considered to be safe for most adults. Side effects occur infrequently, are usually mild, and may include headache, dizziness, and upset stomach. This herb may increase the effects of cardiac glycoside drugs (e.g., digoxin), antihypertensives, and cholesterol-lowering drugs.

Of Special Interest to Women

- There are anecdotal reports that hawthorn can help reduce or eliminate night sweats associated with PMS and menopause. You will likely need to take hawthorn for a month or longer before you will notice results.

• Do not use hawthorn if you are pregnant or breast-feeding, as there is insufficient data on its impact in these situations.

HORSE CHESTNUT

The areas around Greece and Bulgaria are the native home of horse chestnut (*Aesculus hippocastanum*), a tree whose leaves, bark, and flowers have been used for healing purposes for centuries. Today, however, most experts recommend using only the seeds, since the other parts can be toxic if not handled properly. The active ingredient in this herb is called aescin (escin).

Benefits of Horse Chestnut

Much laboratory, animal, and human research has shown that horse chestnut can effectively treat chronic venous insufficiency, a condition in which the veins in the legs do not efficiently return blood to the heart. People with this condition typically have varicose veins and experience pain, itching, leg cramps during sleep, and swollen ankles. Horse chestnut can significantly decrease all of these symptoms. The herb is also used to treat hemorrhoids.

How to Use Horse Chestnut

Look for horse chestnut seed extract that is standardized to contain 16 to 20 percent aescin and is free of aesculin. Supplements are available as capsules and tablets. A typical dose is 300 mg every twelve hours (containing 50 mg of aescin per dose) for up to twelve weeks. Topical forms are available, but they are not effective. Occasionally, horse chestnut can cause nausea, stomach upset, or itching. Do not take nonsteroidal anti-inflammatory drugs (e.g., aspirin, ibuprofen) while using horse chestnut, as this combination may increase the risk of bleeding. Avoid this herb if you have liver or kidney problems.

Of Special Interest to Women

If you are pregnant or breast-feeding, do not use horse chestnut supplements.

PEPPERMINT

Peppermint (*Mentha x piperita*) is a cross between two types of mint (spearmint and water mint) and a plant that is valued for its healing qualities and flavor. Both the essential oils and the leaves of the peppermint plant, which grows throughout North America and Europe, contain menthol, which has soothing, anesthetic properties.

Benefits of Peppermint

Since ancient times, peppermint oil and the leaves have been recognized for their ability to relieve nausea, indigestion, and symptoms related to colds, such as cough, sore throat, and nasal congestion. In more recent years it has proven effective in treating irritable bowel syndrome, because it is a natural antispasmodic that relaxes the smooth muscles in the intestinal tract.

How to Use Peppermint

Peppermint oil is available in bulk, as enteric-coated capsules, as soft gelatin capsules, as lozenges, and in liquid form. Dried peppermint leaves can be used to make tea. Peppermint oil is a potent substance that should always be diluted and used with caution. The typical dose for irritable bowel syndrome and other intestinal and digestion disorders is 0.2 to 0.4 mL of peppermint oil in enteric-coated capsules taken three times daily. To use a liquid form, take 2 to 3 mL of tincture (1:5 in 45 percent ethanol) three times daily, or 1 mL of spirits (10 percent oil and 1 percent leaf extract mixed with water). To make a tea (infusion), use 3 to 6 grams of peppermint leaf steeped for 10 minutes in boiled water.

Enteric-coated capsules help release the oil gradually, greatly reducing the risk of heartburn and nausea. If you take peppermint oil capsules, do not take antacids at the same time, as the medications may break down the coating too quickly and cause side effects.

Of Special Interest to Women

If you are pregnant or breast-feeding, there is only one way you should use peppermint oil: Place a few drops on a handkerchief and inhale the aroma whenever you feel nauseated. Otherwise, do not take peppermint oil internally. For morning sickness, one to two cups of peppermint tea per day is believed to be safe.

PSYLLIUM

Psyllium is derived from the husks of the seeds of *Plantago ovata,* a plant that is native to parts of Asia, the Mediterranean, and North Africa. Today it is cultivated widely in India and Pakistan and in the southwestern United States.

Psyllium contains a high level of soluble fiber (approximately 70 percent soluble fiber and 30 percent insoluble fiber), and the seeds are coated with mucilage, a gummy substance that does not dissolve in water and is not digested by the body. These qualities are the main source of this herb's medicinal powers.

Benefits of Psyllium

Many studies support the ability of psyllium to lower both total cholesterol and low-density lipoprotein (LDL, "bad cholesterol") levels after only eight weeks of daily use. This characteristic has earned psyllium the title of "heart-healthy." Psyllium is effective both as a laxative for treating constipation and as a stool-bulking agent for diarrhea. This may sound contradictory, but in cases of diarrhea, the mucilage absorbs water from the intestines and makes their contents more solid. Psyllium also slows down the stomach and intestines, which allows more water to be reabsorbed, thus controlling diarrhea.

In some studies, psyllium has relieved symptoms of irritable bowel syndrome and inflammatory bowel disease, reduced high blood sugar levels, and helped with weight loss. Researchers are also studying psyllium for possible cancer-fighting effects.

How to Use Psyllium

Psyllium is available in powder, capsules, tablets, and chewable wafers. It is a common ingredient in many over-the-counter laxatives. How much psyllium you need depends on your dietary fiber intake and the condition you want to correct. The recommended daily intake of dietary fiber for adults is 20 to 35 grams daily. Doses of psyllium range from 4 to 20 grams daily as needed (a level teaspoon is about 5 grams). Regardless of the form of psyllium you take, drink lots of water with each dose (at least 8 ounces per 3.5 grams of psyllium). To use the powder, stir it into a glass of water and drink it immediately before it thickens. To avoid gas and bloating, start with a low dose and gradually increase it as your body adjusts to the additional fiber.

Of Special Interest to Women

Psyllium is safe to use if you are pregnant or breastfeeding.

RED CLOVER
Red clover is a perennial herb whose dried red flowers are valued for their medicinal qualities. Its healing abilities

are attributed to isoflavones, plant-based chemicals that have an estrogenlike effect in the body. Red clover is one of the richest sources of isoflavones.

Benefits of Red Clover

A double-blind, placebo-controlled study found that red clover significantly reduced the rate of menopausal symptoms and also lowered triglyceride levels. Researchers also note that the isoflavones in red clover may help relieve hot flashes and diminished memory and cognition associated with menopause, as well as lower cholesterol levels, which may help reduce the risk of cardiovascular disease. One more benefit is suggested by animal studies, which indicate that red clover may increase bone mineral content and help prevent osteoporosis.

How to Use Red Clover

Red clover supplements are available as dried herb (for tea), powdered herb (in capsules), tincture, and fluid extract. A typical dose of the powdered herb is 40 to 160 mg daily, or 28 to 85 mg of red clover isoflavones. If you take the tincture (1:5, 30 percent alcohol), use 60 to 100 drops (3 mL to 5 mL) in water three times daily. The fluid extract (1:1) may also be added to hot water as a tea, 1 mL three times daily. To make tea (infusion), use 1 to 2 teaspoons of dried flowers steeped in 8 ounces of hot water for 30 minutes. Drink two to three cups daily.

Red clover does not appear to cause any serious side effects. Mild reactions may include rash, nausea, or headache. Red clover may alter hormone levels in the body or the effects of any drugs that contain hormones. Talk to your doctor before using red clover if you are taking anticoagulant drugs.

Of Special Interest to Women

Do not use red clover if you are pregnant or breast-feeding.

ST. JOHN'S WORT

St. John's wort (*Hypericum perforatum*) is a shrubby plant that sports yellow flowers and the distinction from ancient times that it could drive out evil spirits, treat nervous conditions, and serve as a balm for burns, wounds, and insect bites. Today St. John's wort is known for its effect on mood and its antibacterial, antiviral, and anti-inflammatory qualities. It is one of the most commonly purchased herbal remedies in the United States.

St. John's wort contains many components, but the ones most studied are hypericin and pseudohypericin. These are found in the flowers and leaves and are believed to be its active ingredients.

Benefits of St. John's Wort

Extensive research on St. John's wort shows that it can reduce depressive symptoms in mild to moderate depression. In fact, it is equally effective as both tricyclic antidepressants and selective serotonin reuptake inhibitors (SSRIs), and has many fewer side effects. Other research indicates that St. John's wort may help relieve symptoms of premenstrual syndrome (e.g., cramping, food cravings, breast tenderness), reduce anxiety, ease hemorrhoids and minor burns (used topically), and fight bacterial infections.

How to Use St. John's Wort

The flowering tops and leaves of St. John's wort are used to make concentrated extracts, which are put into capsules, tablets, tinctures, teas, and oil-based lotions and creams. Look for products that are standardized to contain 0.3% hypericin.

Typical dosing for the dry herb (in tablets or capsules) is 300 to 500 mg three times daily, with meals, for mild depression and mood disorders. If you choose the liquid extract (1:1), take 40 to 60 drops twice a day. To make an infusion, pour 8 ounces of boiling water over 1 to 2 teaspoons of dried herb and steep for 10 minutes. Drink up to two cups daily. If you are treating hemorrhoids, apply the cream or lotion daily. The beneficial effects of oral St. John's wort generally take up to eight weeks to become apparent.

Potential side effects are generally mild and may include rash, fatigue, headache, dry mouth, dizziness, or stomach upset. St. John's wort may cause the skin to become oversensitive to sunlight. To avoid this side effect, use sunscreen while taking St. John's wort.

Of Special Interest to Women

• Until more studies are done, do not use St. John's wort if you are pregnant or breast-feeding.

• Rarely, women who take St. John's wort while using birth control pills experience breakthrough bleeding, as the herb may reduce the effectiveness of the pill.

TEA TREE OIL

Oil derived from the tea tree (*Melaleuca alternifolia;* also known as the ti tree or paperbark tree) has been a part of Australian Aborigine traditional folk medicine for millennia. Captain James Cook named this tree when he discovered that he could use the leaves to make tea. But the therapeutic powers of the oil remained a secret from the world until the 1920s when Australian servicemen discovered that it was a very effective antiseptic for wounds, cuts, and skin infections. The active healing substance is believed to be terpinen-4-ol.

Benefits of Tea Tree Oil

Tea tree oil is effective against various bacteria, viruses, and fungi and is used to treat related skin conditions, including acne, athlete's foot, dandruff, eczema, periodontal disease, toenail fungal infections, vaginitis, and yeast infections. Recent studies suggest tea tree oil may be effective against methicillin-resistant *Staphylococcus aureus* (MRSA), a highly antibiotic-resistant and deadly bacteria.

How to Use Tea Tree Oil

Tea tree oil is available as the oil and in gel or creams. Preparations of the oil come in different strengths, ranging from 5 to 100 percent. For treating acne, the usual strength is 5 to 15 percent; for vaginitis, 1 to 40 percent; and for fungal infections, 70 to 100 percent. The preparation should be applied two to three times daily until symptoms resolve. Because tea tree oil can irritate the skin, it is best to start with a low concentration to determine your tolerance.

Tea tree oil is generally safe when used topically. Occasionally it may cause rash, temporary dryness, itching, redness, irritation, and eczema in people who are allergic to the oil. Tea tree oil should never be taken orally nor used in the ears because it may cause hearing loss.

Of Special Interest to Women

Do not use tea tree oil if you are pregnant or breast-feeding. Some experts recommend avoiding tea tree oil if you have a hormone-related disease, such as breast or ovarian cancer.

UVA URSI

Uva ursi (*Arctostaphylos uva-ursi*), also known as bearberry, is a broadleaf evergreen plant that grows close to the ground and can be found throughout Europe and much of the United States. Traditionally it has been used as an astringent (it causes skin to tighten), to treat diarrhea and dysentery, and for urinary tract infections. Some folk medicine practitioners used it as a remedy for bronchitis.

The main active ingredients in uva ursi are glycoside arbutin and methylarbutin. These components are converted in the intestinal tract into hydroquinone, which is a potent antibacterial agent.

Benefits of Uva Ursi

Uva ursi is an antiseptic that is especially helpful in soothing and strengthening the membranes of the urinary system, including the kidney and bladder. Studies have looked at its ability to treat urinary tract infections, such as cystitis, and thus far this is the main use for this herb.

How to Use Uva Ursi

To make an infusion (tea), pour 8 ounces of boiling water over 1 to 2 teaspoons of dried leaves and let it steep for 10 to 15 minutes. Have three cups per day. If you choose a tincture, take 2 to 5 mL three times daily. Dosage of the capsules or tablets is 250 to 500 mg three times daily. When choosing capsules or tablets, look for those that contain 20 percent arbutin.

Research indicates that uva ursi is much more effective if the urine is alkaline, which can be achieved if you eat a diet that is mainly plant-based. Do not take uva ursi continuously for more than fourteen days. The only side effect associated with uva ursi is mild nausea.

Of Special Interest to Women

Experts do not agree on whether uva ursi is safe to use during pregnancy. Although some experts insist that pregnant women can safely drink two cups of uva ursi tea daily for up to seven days, others recommend avoiding it. Talk to your health care practitioner if you wish to use uva ursi while pregnant or breast-feeding.

VALERIAN

Valerian (*Valeriana officinalis*) is a perennial flowering herb native to Europe and Asia that now grows around the world. It has a long tradition of use for conditions ranging from headache to insomnia, anxiety, digestive disorders, urinary tract infections, angina, and depression. The dried root is believed to contain the herb's active ingredient, which scientists have identified as valerenic acid.

Benefits of Valerian

Several studies in adults indicate that valerian reduces the amount of time it takes to fall asleep and also improves the quality of sleep for up to four to six weeks. In fact, a 2007 study conducted at Emory University in Atlanta, Georgia, investigators found that nearly 6 percent of the more than 31,000 people surveyed said they used valerian root supplements to help them beat insomnia. People who are poor sleepers tend to respond better to valerian than do people who do not have a significant sleep problem. A few studies indicate that valerian may be helpful in relieving anxiety symptoms.

How to Use Valerian

The suggested dose of valerian root extract ranges from 300 to 600 mg, depending on its use, while an equivalent dose of dried root is 2 to 3 g steeped in 8 ounces of hot water for ten to fifteen minutes.

Side effects are rare and may include headache, gastrointestinal distress, or dizziness. People who take high doses of valerian may experience a "hangover" effect, while they may experience withdrawal symptoms (e.g., rapid heartbeat, confusion) if they stop taking the herb suddenly after chronic high-dose use.

Of Special Interest to Women

Do not use valerian root if you are pregnant or breast-feeding, as there is no accurate information about its effect.

AMINO ACIDS AND MISCELLANEOUS SUPPLEMENTS

AMINO ACIDS

Amino acids are the elements that make up proteins. The amino acids discussed here include several that can be helpful for women's health conditions; namely

- Carnitine, an amino acid derivative, is found in nearly every cell in the body.

- Lysine is an essential amino acid, which means the body cannot manufacture it and so you must get it from food.

- Taurine is one of the most abundant amino acids in the body.

- Theanine is related to the amino acid glutamine and is found in tea.

Benefits of Amino Acids

A 2007 study found that carnitine supplements given to women who had fibromyalgia improved their pain, concentration, and quality of life. Carnitine also plays a major role in energy production. Lysine is often used both orally and topically to treat genital herpes and shingles. It helps lower cholesterol, manufacture carnitine, absorb and conserve calcium, and produce energy. Researchers are also considering its effectiveness in relieving migraine symptoms.

Taurine appears to be helpful in treating congestive heart failure and may be beneficial in diabetes, epilepsy, gallbladder disease, and high blood pressure. It also assists the release of neurotransmitters in the brain (which helps mood) and protects cell membranes. Theanine may reduce stress and anxiety and improve mood and cognition. That's because theanine blocks glucocorticoids, stress hormones that are activated by stress and depression.

How to Take Amino Acids

- Carnitine: Daily dose can range from 500 to 2,000 mg, but start with 500 mg, as many people do quite well on this lower dose.

- Lysine: Available in capsules, tablets, liquid, and cream. When used as a preventive for herpes, for example, the dose is 500 to 1,500 mg daily; for active disease, 3,000 to 9,000 mg daily.

- Taurine: Available as a powder and in capsules and tablets. A typical dose is 500 to 1,500 mg daily, but may increase up to 2 g three times daily in some medical conditions.

- Theanine: Take 50 to 200 mg up to three times daily. It can relieve stress and anxiety without causing drowsiness.

Of Special Interest to Women

If you are pregnant or breast-feeding, talk to your doctor before you start taking any amino acid supplement. Amino acids are not harmful to a fetus or nursing infant;

however, maintaining an amino acid balance in the body is necessary for good health, and taking a single amino acid as a supplement may disrupt that balance.

CAROTENOIDS

Carotenoids are the pigments that give plants, including fruits and vegetables, their color. Red peppers, yellow squash, orange carrots, blueberries, and purple eggplant all owe their brilliant colors to carotenoids. Nearly six hundred naturally occurring carotenoids have been discovered thus far. Some of the more common carotenoids are alpha-carotene, beta-carotene, cryptoxanthin, lutein, lycopene, and zeaxanthin.

Benefits of Carotenoids

One of the main functions of certain carotenoids (i.e., alpha-carotene, beta-carotene, cryptoxanthin) is provitamin A activity, which means they convert to vitamin A once they are in the body (see "Vitamin A"). Less than 10 percent of carotenoids have provitamin A activity. Another function of many carotenoids is to act as antioxidants and protect cells, tissues, and organs from free-radical damage. They also inhibit the development of certain types of cancer.

How to Use Carotenoids

Dietary supplements that provide carotenoids individually and in combination are best absorbed if they are taken with a meal that contains fat. The vitamin A activity of beta-carotene in supplements is twice that of beta-carotene that comes from food. That means it takes only 2 mcg of beta-carotene from supplements to provide 1 mcg of retinol (preformed vitamin A). To confuse matters, beta-carotene content in supplements is usually listed in international units (IU) rather than mcg, so use this formula as a guide: 3,000 mcg (3 mg) of beta-carotene provides 5,000 IU of vitamin A.

Lycopene, lutein, and zeaxanthin are available as individual supplements. Lutein and zeaxanthin are often combined in a single product.

Of Special Interest to Women

Unlike vitamin A, high doses of beta-carotene taken by pregnant women have not been linked to an increased risk of birth defects. Although there appears to be no reason to restrict use of beta-carotene during pregnancy or breastfeeding, women in these situations should take no more than 3 mg/day (5,000 IU/day) of beta-carotene from supplements unless instructed otherwise by their doctor. Other carotenoid supplements are also likely safe in pregnancy and lactation, but they should be avoided simply as a precaution.

COENZYME Q_{10}

Coenzyme Q_{10} (coQ_{10}) is a vitamin-like substance produced by the human body. It is found in the energy-producing part of cells (the mitochondria) and participates in the manufacture of ATP, the main energy source of cells. CoQ_{10} also is a potent antioxidant and helps destroy free radicals that can damage the body.

Scientists know that levels of coQ_{10} decline with age and that low levels are found in people who have various chronic diseases, such as heart disease, cancer, and diabetes. In some cases, coQ_{10} supplementation may help in the treatment of such conditions.

Benefits of CoQ_{10}

Many of the benefits associated with coQ_{10} are related to the heart. Studies show, for example, that people who took coQ_{10} daily within three days of having a heart attack were significantly less likely to have a subsequent heart attack or chest pain. CoQ_{10} may reduce leg swelling and improve breathing in people who have congestive heart failure, and it may also lower blood pressure. Some evidence indicates that it could help with headache, fibromyalgia, and ovarian cancer.

How to Use CoQ$_{10}$

CoQ$_{10}$ is available in capsules and tablets and as an oral spray. The typical dose is 50 to 150 mg daily for high blood pressure or congestive heart failure, and 120 mg daily for four weeks after experiencing a heart attack. Take coQ$_{10}$ with a meal that contains some fat so your body can adequately absorb the supplement.

CoQ$_{10}$ occasionally can cause mild, brief side effects, including nausea, vomiting, heartburn, diarrhea, insomnia, loss of appetite, rash, headache, dizziness, and irritability. Because coQ$_{10}$ may lower blood sugar levels, use it with caution if you have hypoglycemia or diabetes or are taking drugs or supplements that affect blood sugar.

Of Special Interest to Women

- Because the safety of coQ$_{10}$ during pregnancy and breast-feeding is not known, it is best to avoid this supplement during these times.

- Although evidence is limited, several studies suggest that coQ$_{10}$ may help prevent recurrence or metastasis of breast cancer.

DHEA

Dehydroepiandrosterone (DHEA) is a steroid hormone that is secreted by the adrenal gland. It is often called the "mother of all hormones" because it is the precursor to male and female sex hormones; that is, DHEA is converted into estrogen and other sex hormones. Levels of DHEA begin to decrease in everyone after age 30, but low levels are routinely also seen in people who have adrenal insufficiency, anorexia, type 2 diabetes, depression, lupus, and other chronic conditions.

Benefits of DHEA

Several small but promising studies indicate that DHEA may improve hormone levels, quality of life, and general well-being in people who have adrenal insufficiency. Many of the clinical trials that have used DHEA to treat depression, lupus, and obesity have also had positive results. Less convincing are studies of DHEA in Alzheimer's disease, bone loss, cardiovascular disease, infertility, and fibromyalgia.

How to Use DHEA

Generally, DHEA is not recommended for people who are younger than 40 unless they have abnormally low levels (<130 mg/dL for women, <180 mg/dL for men). Have your DHEA levels checked (with a blood test) before starting a supplement program.

DHEA is available in capsules and tablets. Women generally respond best to doses between 5 and 25 mg per day, although up to 50 mg may be necessary in some cases of adrenal insufficiency or anorexia. The best time to take DHEA is in the early morning because that is when the body produces it naturally.

Of Special Interest to Women

Taking DHEA supplements can cause levels of estrogens and androgens to rise, which may increase the risk of hormone-related cancers (e.g., breast, ovarian, cervical). DHEA supplements also cause some women to experience deepening of the voice, development of facial hair, acne, hair loss, and oily skin. Its use has also been associated with a rise in blood sugar levels, altered thyroid hormone levels, and changes in cholesterol levels. Therefore, DHEA should be taken only under a doctor's supervision.

5-HTP

5-hydroxytryptophan (5-HTP) is an amino acid that is the intermediate step between tryptophan (an amino acid) and its conversion to the brain chemical serotonin. Low serotonin levels are associated with depression, cravings for carbohydrates, frequent headaches, being overweight, and muscle pain. If you have low 5-HTP levels, then low serotonin levels usually are not far behind.

5-HTP occurs naturally in two places—in the human body and in the seeds of the *Griffonia simplicifolia* plant, which is a native of west Africa. Extracts of these seeds are used to make 5-HTP supplements.

Benefits of 5-HTP

Because 5-HTP converts to serotonin, 5-HTP supplements allow you to enjoy the same benefits you would get if you could take serotonin supplements—improved mood, better sleep, appetite suppression, relief from muscle aches and pains, and feeling of calm. However, because serotonin supplements are not available, 5-HTP is the most direct way to boost the levels of this brain chemical.

How to Use 5-HTP

5-HTP is available in capsules and caplets. The typical dose is 25 to 50 mg daily. Because 5-HTP makes some people feel sleepy (which is appropriate if you take it for insomnia), it may be best to take it at night before retiring.

Side effects are generally mild and may include stomach cramps, nausea, and nightmares. Use of medications that affect serotonin levels (e.g., selective serotonin

reuptake inhibitors, triptans) along with 5-HTP may increase the risk of developing serotonin syndrome, a rare
but serious condition characterized by confusion, muscle
rigidity, blood pressure changes, and coma.

Of Special Interest to Women

Use of 5-HTP during pregnancy and breast-feeding cannot be recommended because of a lack of scientific information. Use of 5-HTP may suppress lactation.

GLUCOSAMINE

Glucosamine is a natural substance, made from the amino
acid glutamine and glucose, that is found in healthy cartilage. Its job is to stimulate the formation and repair of joint
cartilage. Glucosamine production slows with age.

Glucosamine supplements are sold alone or combined
with another natural substance called chondroitin sulfate.
Chondroitin is a major component of cartilage, and its main
function is to maintain the structure of joint cartilage by
preventing body enzymes from breaking it down.

Benefits of Glucosamine

Studies show that glucosamine sulfate may relieve symptoms of mild to moderate osteoarthritis of the knee, including inflammation and pain. Glucosamine sulfate may also
improve pain, mobility, and swelling in osteoarthritis of
other joints, although fewer studies have been done. Preliminary studies are exploring whether glucosamine may
be helpful in rheumatoid arthritis and inflammatory bowel
disease.

How to Use Glucosamine

Glucosamine sulfate is available as capsules, tablets, and
powder. The typical dose is 500 mg of glucosamine sulfate

three times daily for thirty to ninety days. Some experts recommend taking 20 mg per kg (2.2 pounds) of body weight daily, in divided doses.

Glucosamine may cause minor side effects, including drowsiness, insomnia, headache, sun sensitivity, and toughening of the nails. In theory, glucosamine may reduce the effectiveness of insulin or other drugs or herbs used to control blood glucose levels. It is also possible that glucosamine may increase the risk of bleeding when it is taken with drugs that pose the same risk (e.g., aspirin, ibuprofen, heparin).

Because glucosamine supplements may be made from the shells of shellfish, do not use these supplements if you have a shellfish allergy or are hypersensitive to iodine.

Of Special Interest to Women

Glucosamine cannot be recommended during pregnancy or breast-feeding because of the lack of scientific evidence.

MELATONIN

Melatonin is a neurohormone manufactured in the brain by the pineal gland. Production and release of this hormone follow a set pattern: They are stimulated by darkness and inhibited by light, which indicates that this hormone is involved in the body's circadian rhythm and sleep patterns.

Benefits of Melatonin

Melatonin is used successfully to treat insomnia and jet lag. Many studies have shown that melatonin taken 30 to 120 minutes before retiring decreases the amount of time it takes to fall asleep.

Scientists are also investigating whether melatonin may be effective in many other disorders, including cancer, glaucoma, headache, high blood pressure, and Parkinson's disease, among others.

How to Use Melatonin

Melatonin supplements can be either synthetic or natural. The natural form is made from the pineal gland of animals and carries the risk of viral contamination; thus the synthetic form is recommended.

Low doses (0.1 to 0.3 mg per night) appear to be just as effective as higher doses (3 to 5 mg per night) among both young, healthy adults and the elderly, so start with a low dose and increase it as needed. Some research indicates that quick-release formulas are more effective than sustained-release forms, yet a 2007 study in the *Journal of Sleep Research* found that the sustained form improved both quality of sleep and morning alertness in people 55 and older.

Side effects associated with melatonin include headache, stomach discomfort, depression, or feeling hung over. Because there is a risk of daytime sleepiness when taking melatonin, you should know how you respond to this hormone before you drive or engage in potentially dangerous activities.

Of Special Interest to Women

Women who are pregnant or attempting to get pregnant should avoid using melatonin because it may alter the function of the pituitary gland and affect ovulation or uterine contractions. High levels of melatonin during pregnancy may increase the risk of developmental disorders.

MSM

Methylsulfonylmethane (MSM) is a naturally occurring nutrient present in small amounts in many foods. It provides sulfur, a vital substance that is a component of joints, cartilage, skin, hair, and nails, and is essential to support many biochemical processes in the body, including energy production. As a dietary supplement, MSM is synthesized to mimic the natural product.

Benefits of MSM

MSM is used to relieve pain and inflammation associated with various conditions, including arthritis, back pain, fibromyalgia, lupus, and pelvic inflammatory disease, which it does by inhibiting the actions of substances that cause inflammation (e.g., prostaglandins and leukotrienes). Its high sulfur content (34 percent) is key in its ability to help maintain the health of cartilage, skin, nails, and hair. The sulfur content of cartilage declines with age, and that decline parallels the deterioration of the joints; thus supplementation with MSM appears to be a way to prevent further deterioration and perhaps replenish the sulfur in the joints.

How to Use MSM

MSM is available in capsules, tablets, and powder. A typical daily dose ranges from 1,500 to 6,000 mg. Because MSM may increase your energy level, avoid taking it before retiring, always split the dose, and take it with meals. Side effects are mild and infrequent and may include loose stools or headache.

Of Special Interest to Women

MSM use cannot be recommended during pregnancy or breast-feeding because of the lack of scientific evidence.

SAM-E

S-adenosyl-L-methionine (SAM-e) is formed from methionine, an amino acid, and adenosine triphosphate (ATP), an element that is involved in energy production. SAM-e is found in every cell in the body and contributes to more than a hundred different reactions. It plays an important role in the formation, activation, or metabolism of hormones, proteins, fats, and neurotransmitters.

Benefits of SAM-e

Studies show that SAM-e can relieve symptoms of depression, osteoarthritis, and liver disease. For depression, SAM-e is necessary in the production and activity of brain chemicals that improve mood (e.g., the neurotransmitters dopamine and serotonin). When compared with various antidepressant drugs, SAM-e provides faster results and is better tolerated.

SAM-e can improve joint health by protecting the joints and increasing the formation of cartilage. It also reduces inflammation and pain. In the liver, SAM-e helps remove toxins and improve the flow of bile.

How to Use SAM-e

SAM-e is available in tablets and capsules. Dosing depends on the condition you are treating. Typical dosing for depression and osteoarthritis begins at 400 mg and increases over time, while dosing for fibromyalgia and liver disorders tends to start lower.

You can expect best results if you take SAM-e on an empty stomach, but if you experience stomach irritation, take it with meals. Because the body naturally has higher SAM-e levels during the day, avoid taking it at night.

SAM-e may trigger a manic phase in people who have bipolar disorder. It also should not be used if you have Parkinson's disease.

Of Special Interest to Women

SAM-e is sometimes used to treat a condition called cholestasis, a common liver disease that happens only during pregnancy. In cholestasis, the normal flow of bile in the gallbladder is disrupted by the high levels of pregnancy hormones in the body. The bile builds up in the liver and spills into the bloodstream. Often the only symptom is intense itching of the hands and/or feet, but depression, loss of appetite, and fatigue may occur as well. Cholestasis may increase the risk for preterm birth, stillbirth, or fetal distress. Cholestasis disappears after delivery.

PART III
Your Personal Supplement Plan

In this section we explain how to build a personal supplement program that fits your unique needs. One important thing you need to understand before we go any further is that the most wonderful supplement program in the world cannot replace or be a substitute for a basic foundation for health. That foundation should be built on four pillars: a nutritional diet, adequate sleep, regular exercise, and basic healthy lifestyle choices (e.g., stress management, no smoking, reasonable alcohol use). A supplement program enhances that foundation, providing you with extra boosts that can help you maintain a state of wellness, prevent infections and disease, and, if necessary, treat any medical conditions that develop. A personal supplement program can improve your physical, emotional, and spiritual well-being and allow you the flexibility to make changes when your needs change as you age, begin new life stages (e.g., pregnancy, breastfeeding, menopause), or face new challenges (e.g., recovery from surgery, development of chronic disease).

You can create your own personal supplement program in three simple steps. (The fourth step is really a revisit to step 2, and it only comes into play when there is a life-changing event.)

- Step 1: Choose a high-quality multivitamin/mineral based on your dietary habits.

• Step 2: Evaluate your unique nutritional needs.

• Step 3: Be a knowledgeable shopper.

• Step 4: Reevaluate your supplement needs when a life-changing situation arises.

You don't have to do this alone: We provide some guidelines and questions for each step so you can easily make your selections. As a general rule, consult with your health care practitioner before beginning a supplement program.

STEP 1: CHOOSE A MULTIVITAMIN/MINERAL

The number of multivitamin/mineral supplements on the market claiming to be the "perfect" one for you is staggering. Obviously all of them can't be right for you, but with a little effort you can find the ones that fit your needs, based on your dietary habits. So let's look at those habits for a moment.

Do you eat a lot of whole foods—fresh fruits and vegetables, whole grains and whole-grain products, and beans and legumes? Do you limit your fat intake to less than 30 percent? If this sounds like you, a supplement that provides doses at the lower end of the ranges is probably sufficient for you.

Do you frequent fast-food restaurants, eat lots of processed foods at home, and use your vegetable crisper to store bottles of soda? Then you should choose a multivitamin/mineral that provides doses at the higher end of the ranges.

Regardless of which multiple product you choose, you will likely need to take a separate supplement for calcium, as women generally need much more of this mineral than is found in a multiple supplement. If your health care practitioner has determined that you need iron, you may want to choose a supplement that provides this mineral, or you may elect to take a separate supplement.

The multiple you choose should contain all of the vitamins and minerals listed in Table I and provide doses that fall within the safe, recommended ranges listed. When you go shopping, some of the supplements you see may contain very small amounts of trace minerals such as silica, vanadium, and iodine. These ingredients are not necessary, so do not be concerned if the supplement you choose does not have these nutrients.

Here are a few other things to consider when looking for and taking a multivitamin/mineral.

- Once-a-day or several-a-day? Once-a-day multiples are convenient, especially for people who have trouble remembering to take pills. Multiples that are designed to be taken in two or more dosages throughout the day, however, are usually better absorbed and allow you the flexibility to change the amount of supplement you take based on the quality of your diet on any given day.

- Always take your multivitamin/mineral with a meal because your body is better able to assimilate the nutrients. Taking a multiple supplement on an empty stomach also can cause queasiness or nausea in some people.

- Do not take your supplement with coffee or tea.

STEP 2: EVALUATE YOUR UNIQUE NUTRITIONAL NEEDS

Now it's time to individualize your program by identifying any special nutritional needs related to your lifestyle and health or medical conditions so you can determine which nutrients you need to address those issues. Do you have a history of heart disease in your family? Then you may want to include coenzyme Q_{10} or hawthorn as part of your supplement program. Do you have insomnia? Then extra magnesium may be helpful. Are you pregnant or

TABLE I

NUTRIENT	RECOMMENDED RANGE
Vitamins	
Vitamin A (as retinol)	2,500–5,000 IU[1]
Beta-carotene	5,000–25,000 IU
Vitamin B_1	10–100 mg
Vitamin B_2 (riboflavin)	10–50 mg
Vitamin B_3 (niacin/niacinamide)	10–100 mg/10–30 mg
Vitamin B_5 (pantothenic acid)	25–100 mg
Vitamin B_6 (pyridoxine)	25–100 mg
Biotin	100–600 mcg
Folic acid	400–800 mcg
Vitamin B_{12}	400 mcg
Vitamin C	250–500 mg
Vitamin D	100–400 IU
Vitamin E	100–400 IU
Choline	10–100 mg
Minerals	
Calcium	250–1,000 mg[2]
Chromium	200–400 mcg
Copper	1–2 mg
Iron	15–30 mg[3]
Magnesium	250–350 mg
Manganese	10–15 mg
Molybdenum	10–25 mcg
Selenium	100–200 mcg
Zinc	15–20 mg

1. Women of childbearing age should not take more than 2,500 IU of vitamin A (as retinol) daily, as there is an increased risk of birth defects at higher amounts.
2. Calcium is best taken as a separate supplement, so don't worry about how much is in your multiple.
3. Choose a multiple with iron only if your doctor has determined that you need iron.

planning to get pregnant soon? Then you need to pay attention to your folic acid intake.

Here is a checklist of statements you can review to help you choose which natural supplements you may want to add to your basic multivitamin/mineral supplement. For every yes answer, you can refer to the associated entry in Part I to read more about which supplements you may want to add to your personal supplement program. (For example, for the statement "I am going through menopause," refer to the entry for "Menopause.")

Health/Medical Conditions

- I have acne.

- I am fatigued much of the time (see "Adrenal Fatigue," "Anemia," "Chronic Fatigue Syndrome," "Fibromyalgia," "Lupus").

- My menstrual cycle has stopped (see "Amenorrhea," "Menopause").

- I have anemia.

- I have an eating disorder (see "Anorexia Nervosa").

- I am overly anxious and/or I have panic attacks.

- I have asthma.

- I have back pain.

- I have a history of breast cancer in my family/I have breast cancer.

- I have numbness, pain, and/or tingling in my hands/I have carpal tunnel syndrome.

- I have a history of cervical cancer in my family/I have cervical cancer.

- I have chlamydia.

- I have constipation/I have a tendency to be constipated.

- I am sad and/or depressed.

- I have a history of diabetes in my family/I have diabetes or prediabetes.

- My eyes are abnormally dry (see "Dry Eye Syndrome").

- I have a history of endometrial cancer in my family/I have endometrial cancer.

- I have tender/painful lumps in my breasts (see "Fibrocystic Breast Changes").

- I have fibromyalgia.

- I have a history of gallstones in my family/I have gallstones.

- I am losing my hair.

- I experience frequent headache/migraine.

- I have a history of heart disease in my family/I have heart disease.

- I have hemorrhoids.

- I have herpes.

- I have high blood pressure.

- I have hypothyroidism.

- I have urinary incontinence (see "Incontinence").

- I've been unable to get pregnant for a year or longer (see "Infertility").

- I have sleep problems/insomnia.

- I have irritable bowel syndrome/I have chronic problems with diarrhea and constipation.

- I have lupus.

- I am going through menopause.

- I have morning sickness.

- I am overweight/I can't lose weight (see "Obesity").

- I have arthritis (see "Osteoarthritis," "Rheumatoid Arthritis").

- I have a history of ovarian cancer in my family/I have ovarian cancer.

- I have pelvic inflammatory disease.

- I have PMS.

- I have scleroderma.

- I have shingles.

- I have temporomandibular joint disease.

- I am susceptible to urinary tract infections/I have a urinary tract infection.

- I have a yeast infection/I have vaginitis (see "Vaginitis").

- I have varicose veins.

- I have abnormal vaginal discharge (see "Chlamydia," "Pelvic Inflammatory Disease," "Vaginitis").

Lifestyle Factors

- I am lactose-intolerant. (You may need to take additional calcium.)

- I am a strict vegetarian (vegan). (You may need additional vitamin B_{12} and calcium.)

- I am on a very low-calorie diet. (You should take a multivitamin/mineral with values at the high end of the range, plus you may need additional calcium, vitamin E, vitamin B_6, and zinc because of poor nutritional intake.)

- I smoke. (Smokers often need additional antioxidants; see Table II.)

- I am pregnant or planning to get pregnant. (Pregnant women need additional amounts of nearly all nutrients, but you should be especially careful to get enough folic acid and vitamin B_6.)

- I consume alcohol regularly. (If you drink a great deal of alcohol, you may have difficulty absorbing many nutrients, especially the B vitamins; see Table II.)

TABLE II

DRUG	NUTRIENT DEFICIENCY
Alcohol	Vitamins A, B_1, and B_2, biotin, choline, niacin, folic acid, magnesium
Antacids (containing aluminum and calcium)	Phosphorus, vitamin B_1, iron
Anticoagulants	Vitamins A and K
Antihistamines	Vitamin C
Antiseizure drugs and sedatives	Calcium, folic acid, vitamins D and K
Barbiturates	Vitamins A, C, and D, folic acid
Birth control pills and estrogen replacement	Folic acid, vitamin B_6
Caffeine	Vitamins B_1, B_{12}, C, and E; calcium, iron, potassium, zinc
Cimetidine	Vitamin B_1
Diuretics (non-potassium-sparing)	Potassium, magnesium, B complex
Laxatives	Calcium, phosphorus, vitamins A, D, E, and K
Neomycin, cholestyramine	Vitamins A, D, E, K, and B_{12}
Nicotine	Vitamins C, and B_1, folic acid, calcium
Penicillin (all forms)	Niacin, vitamins B_6 and K
Steroids	Vitamins B_6, C, and D
Tetracyclines	Vitamin K, calcium, magnesium, iron

- I take over-the-counter and/or prescription medications. (If you are using any of the drugs listed in Table II in high doses or for a prolonged period of time, you may need additional nutrients.)

If you answered yes to more than one statement in the checklist on pages 233–237, see if any of the suggested supplements provide multiple benefits. For example, if you are battling depression and insomnia, you could choose to take SAM-e for depression and melatonin for insomnia. Or you could choose to take 5-HTP because it has proven to be effective for treating both conditions. Why take two when one will do? You can save both money and time.

One word of caution: Keep track of your add-on supplements. If your multivitamin/mineral provides 10 mg of zinc, for example, and you take an additional 30 mg of zinc to fight a cold and 20 mg more because you know it helps prevent macular degeneration, you will be taking too much zinc, which can impair iron absorption.

STEP 3: BE A KNOWLEDGEABLE SHOPPER

Now you have a list of supplements that fit your unique needs, and so you're ready to shop. But where should you begin? A visit to your favorite pharmacy, nutrition store, or supplement Web site can make your head spin. So many options! So many formulas! So many brands! Which ones are right for you? How do you know if you're getting quality ingredients?

We answer these and related questions in this section. We begin by looking at how to read a supplement label and then offer information on the various forms of natural supplements and how to use them.

How to Read Supplement Labels

Supplement manufacturers have the daunting task of squeezing lots of information into a small space. As a consumer, you have the equally daunting task of reading and interpreting that information. In this section we help you do just that.

Even though dietary supplements are not subjected to the same stringent rules under which drugs are regulated by the Food and Drug Administration (FDA), they must adhere to certain rules when it comes to labeling. In March 1999, new rules concerning the labeling of dietary supplements went into effect. Here's a brief rundown of the information you should see on supplement labels and what it means.

- *Supplement Facts panel (or ingredient statement).* All ingredients must be named in either a Supplement Facts panel/box or an ingredients list.

- *Daily Value (DV).* Daily Value is a dosage recommendation standard that is based on DRIs (Dietary Reference Intakes; see the box on page 240 for explanation). Manufacturers must give the DV recommendations where a reference has been established. For example, a supplement that contains 2 mg of vitamin B_6 per dose would give the DV as 100%. For ingredients without an established DV (e.g., amino acids, herbs), the quantity must be listed and identified as having no DV.

- *Herbs.* All herbs must be identified by their common name and the part of the plant that was used to make the supplement (e.g., root, berries, leaves).

- *Proprietary blends.* These are manufacturers' "secret formulas," and supplement producers are allowed to give the weight for the total blend only. When this is done, the ingredients in the blend must be listed in descending order of predominance by weight.

- *High potency.* When this term is used, it describes a nutrient when it is present at 100 percent or more of the RDA for the specific vitamin or mineral. The term may be used also in multi-ingredient products if two-thirds of the nutrients in the supplement are present at levels that are more than 100 percent of the RDA.

FROM RDAs TO DRIs

From 1941 until 1989, the RDA—the Recommended Daily Allowance—was the standard by which professionals and consumers could decide if they were meeting nutritional requirements to prevent diseases that can be caused by deficiencies. Then in 1997, the Food and Nutrition Board of the National Academy of Sciences created the Dietary References Intakes, or DRIs. These new reference value categories were designed not only to prevent nutrient deficiencies but also to reduce the risk of chronic diseases such as cardiovascular disease, cancer, diabetes, and osteoporosis. The four types of DRI values are explained here. You may see these values when shopping for or reading about supplements.

- *RDA.* The average daily dietary intake level that meets the nutrient needs of 97 to 98 percent of healthy individuals of a specific gender and in a specific stage of life.

- *AI (Adequate Intake).* The recommended intake value based on observations or experimentally determined estimates of the nutrient intake by a group of healthy individuals. This value is used when an RDA cannot be determined.

- *UL (Tolerable Upper Intake Level).* The highest level of daily nutrient intake that is likely to cause no risk to health for nearly all individuals in the general population.

- *EAR (Estimated Average Requirement).* A daily nutrient intake value that is estimated to meet the requirement of half of the healthy people of a specific gender and in a specific life stage.

These guidelines provide a *starting point* for health professionals and consumers alike. In reality, the recommended therapeutic doses of nutrients often far exceed the established DRIs. One good example is vitamin C: Although the DRI for women is 75 mg daily, many people take vitamin C supplements that total 500 mg or more daily. The UL for vitamin C is 2,000 mg, although many people tolerate and reportedly benefit from higher doses. Therefore the important take-home message here is to treat the DRIs as a pivotal point from which you can establish values that fit your own personal needs.

• *Antioxidants.* This term may be used along with the terms "good source" and "high" to describe a nutrient for which there is scientific evidence that taking a sufficient amount of it will disarm free radicals or prevent free-radical-initiated chemical reactions in the body.

• *Provider information.* Labels must provide the name and place of business of the manufacturer, packer, or distributor.

• *Structure-function claims.* These are statements claiming that the supplement can maintain healthy or normal structures or functions of the human body. For example, a fiber supplement may claim that it "maintains bowel regularity." Such statements must be accompanied by a statement that the claim "has not been evaluated by the Food and Drug Administration. This product is not intended to diagnose, treat, cure, or prevent any disease."

- *Expiration date.* This is the date after which a supplement may no longer contain the potency listed on the label. Not all supplements have an expiration date, and for some the date is only an estimate. The truth is, the shelf life for some substances is not yet well known. You can contact the manufacturer or dealer to learn more about how an expiration date was determined or why one was not provided.

- *Lot numbers.* Lot numbers allow you to trace a product through the supply process so the origin of its ingredients can be identified. This is helpful if a product is recalled.

- *Certification.* Most supplements carry a type of "seal of approval" indicating that the product meets the requirements of a specific certification program. Here are just a few of those programs.

  - USP (United States Pharmacopeia) insignia means the manufacturer claims their ingredients have an FDA-approved or USP-accepted use, have been used without significant safety risk, and meet the standards of the USP regarding rates of dissolution, strength, range of acceptable impurities, and expiration date. Manufacturers who have the words "USP Verified" on their label have voluntarily asked the US Pharmacopeia to test their products for identity, potency, and purity, and to review their manufacturing processes. To see a complete list of products that are verified by the USP, see ww.usp.org/USPVerified/dietarySupplements/supplements.

  - NF (National Formulary) insignia means the manufacturer claims that their herbal ingredients have been used without significant safety risk and meet the standards of the USP National Formulary (similar to those above). NF products are not required to have an FDA-approved or USP-accepted use.

You can learn whether the supplements you want to buy contain the ingredients and dosages stated by the manufacturers by checking with ConsumerLab, (www.consumerlab.com), a provider of independent test results and information on nutritional products. ConsumerLab has tested products representing more than 350 different brands and provides their results online.

A few other terms you may see on your supplement labels need to be explained.

- *Other ingredients.* Extra ingredients, called excipients—nonactive ingredients essential to the manufacturing process—are often added to fill space, add flavor or color, bind or stabilize the ingredients, or help prevent manufacturing machinery from clogging. Many supplement manufacturers make a point of listing ingredients that they have *not* added, such as eggs, gluten, milk/lactose, wheat, soy, corn, starch, and yeast. This is important because some people are allergic to these substances. Some excipients may include the following:

- *Magnesium stearate.* An anti-caking substance that makes it easier to encapsulate dry ingredients

- *Gelatin.* A collagen protein used in capsule production

- *Glycerin.* Usually used to make soft gelatin capsules

- *Dicalcium phosphate.* A mixture of calcium and phosphate used as a filler and/or binding agent

- *Stearic acid.* A fatty acid derived from vegetable oils used as a lubricant

- *Chelated minerals.* A chelated mineral is one in which the mineral is bound to a protein molecule. It is believed that chelated minerals are better absorbed by the body and that they cause less gastrointestinal distress.

- *Antioxidants.* Antioxidants are substances that protect your cells against the damage caused by free radicals—molecules that are produced as your body metabolizes food or when you are exposed to toxins from the environment, including but not limited to tobacco smoke, food preservatives, radiation, pesticides, heavy

MEASUREMENT MADNESS

Some dosage units can be confusing. For liquids, dosages are usually given in milliliters (mL) or cubic centimeters (cc). Pills, capsules, powders, and other dry products are given in micrograms (mcg), milligrams (mg), or grams (g). The International Unit (IU) is used for fat-soluble vitamins (A, D, and E) and some hormones and enzymes. Sometimes the values of these vitamins are given in other units of measure, which means you need to know the equivalent amount. Here are the equivalents for the three fat-soluble vitamins:

- Beta-carotene (vitamin A): 1 mg = 833 IU

- Vitamin D: 2.5 mcg = 100 IU

- Vitamin E: 1 mg = 1 IU

metals, and most medications. Antioxidants help prevent cell damage by slowing or preventing oxidation. The cell damage caused by free radicals can lead to cancer, heart disease, liver and kidney disease, and many other serious conditions. Antioxidants may also improve immune system function and thus help reduce your risk for infection.

How to Buy Herbs

When you buy herbal supplements (and when you read the herbal entries in this book), you will often see the words "standardized," "standardized extract," or "guaranteed potency extract." These phrases mean that the manufacturer has verified that the active ingredient in the herb is also present in the herbal supplement at the potency and amount stated on the label. Not all manufacturers standardize their supplements to the same substances, and in some cases there is more than one compound that is active in the herb. A good example is St. John's wort. Several substances appear to be active, including hypericin, which is standardized to 0.3 percent, and hyperforin, standardized to 2 to 5 percent. We have included standardization information for each herb when known.

Herbs are available in a variety of forms, some of which may be unfamiliar to you. Not all herbs are available in every configuration. Here's a breakdown of the more common forms.

- *Tablets and capsules.* These forms contain the dry extract (see "Extract"). Some manufacturers make vegetarian capsules, which means they do not contain gelatin or other animal products.

- *Extract.* Made by soaking the herb in a liquid that removes specific chemicals. The liquid is then used as is or it is evaporated to make a dry extract that is put into capsules and tablets.

- *Tincture.* Made by soaking an herb in a solution of alcohol and water. Tinctures are prepared in different strengths that are expressed as a ratio of herb to extract (i.e., ratios of the weight of the dried herb to the volume or weight of the finished product). To take a tincture, add the recommended number of drops to water and drink it.

- *Tea/infusion.* An infusion is made by adding boiling water to fresh or dried herbs (usually the leaves) and steeping them for ten to twenty minutes. It can be drunk either hot or cold.

- *Decoction.* A decoction is similar to a tea except it is made with the parts of the herb that require more vigorous treatment (e.g., roots, rhizomes, berries, bark) to extract the desired ingredients. These herb parts are usually simmered for at least thirty minutes to prepare a decoction.

RECIPES FOR SUCCESS
Some natural supplements can be used in beverages or food to make taking them more enjoyable. Here are a few simple recipes and tips on ways to use selected natural supplements.

Herbal Infusions

To make a large batch of an herbal infusion, place 1 ounce (approximately 1 cup loosely packed) of dried herb leaves in a 1-quart jar. Fill the jar to the top with boiling water and cap it. Allow the infusion to brew for at least four hours. Strain and drink the recommended number of cups per day.

Flaxseed Dressing
4 tablespoons apple cider vinegar
3–5 tablespoons flaxseed oil
6 tablespoons water
20 almonds

1 tablespoon ground flaxseed
2 teaspoon sea salt
2 tablespoons maple syrup
Crushed black pepper, basil, and thyme to taste

Place all ingredients except the herbs into a blender and process until smooth. Stir in the herbs and chill or use at room temperature.

Flaxseed Smoothie
　1 cup orange juice
　1 cup frozen unsweetened strawberries
　1 banana
　2 tablespoons ground flaxseed

Place all ingredients in a blender and process until smooth.

Flaxseed Cereal
　5 tablespoons flaxseeds
　Cinnamon to taste
　Pinch of salt
　Warm water
　Honey if desired

Blend the flaxseed in a coffee grinder until it is a fine texture. Put into a bowl with the cinnamon and salt. Add warm water until the mixture is creamy. Stir in honey if desired.

Roasted Garlic
　4 heads of garlic
　½ cup vegetable broth
　2 tablespoons margarine, melted
　½ teaspoon thyme
　¼ teaspoon black pepper
　¼ teaspoon salt

Remove the outer papery covering from the garlic but leave the coverings on the individual cloves. Place the heads in a baking dish and dab each with melted margarine. Sprinkle the bulbs with thyme, pepper, and salt. Pour the broth into the dish. Cover the dish with foil and bake at 350° F for 45 minutes, basting frequently. Uncover the dish and bake for another 15 minutes. To serve, separate the garlic head into individual cloves. You can squeeze out the softened garlic from each clove as desired, or squeeze out all the cloves into a serving dish, cover with olive oil, and store tightly covered in the refrigerator for up to one month.

Candied Ginger for Nausea or Morning Sickness
　3 cups water
　1 cup peeled and thinly sliced ginger
　1 cup sugar (or see variation below)

In a saucepan, boil the water. Add the ginger and sugar and cover. Reduce the heat and allow it to simmer for 5 minutes. Remove from heat and let it sit for 20 minutes. Heat the oven to 200° F. Place the ginger slices on a flat baking sheet and place it in the oven. Leave the slices in the oven until they are nearly dry but still chewy. Toss the cooled ginger in sugar to coat. Store the ginger in an airtight container, where it should keep for up to two months.

Variation: If you don't want to use sugar, you can cook the ginger in plain water and coat it in stevia.

Cinnamon to the Rescue

Here are some traditional remedies that have stood the test of time.

- *Cold remedy.* Simmer 1 broken-up cinnamon stick, 1 ounce sliced fresh ginger, 1 teaspoon coriander seeds, 3 cloves, 1 lemon slice, and 16 ounces of water for 15 minutes and then strain. Drink one cup hot every two hours.

- *Diarrhea remedy.* If you risk dehydration, make cinnamon tea by mixing 1 tablespoon of dried powdered cinnamon bark in 8 ounces of hot water. Steep for 10 minutes and then drink.

- *Irregular periods, PMS.* Use the diarrhea remedy twice a day for heavy bleeding or to alleviate cramping and abdominal pain.

- *Gas/bloating.* Use ½ teaspoon ground cinnamon and ½ teaspoon ground ginger in 1 cup of boiling water. Allow to steep for 15 minutes, strain, and drink after each meal.

GLOSSARY

ANTIOXIDANTS: Compounds that prevent damage to cells from oxidation or from molecules known as free radicals. The body can make its own antioxidants but relies heavily on antioxidants from the diet. Dietary antioxidants include vitamins C and E, beta-carotene, selenium, copper, zinc, and phytonutrients.

ATP (adenosine triphosphate)**:** A compound, found in all cells, that is the main energy source for all cell reactions in the body.

BETA-CAROTENE: A type of carotenoid and a plant pigment that is converted into vitamin A in the body. It is also known as provitamin A.

BIOFLAVONOIDS: Compounds found in fruits that contain vitamin C. They are sometimes included in vitamin C supplements.

CAROTENOIDS: Fat-soluble plant pigments that the body converts into vitamin A.

CHELATED: When minerals are bound to proteins, which increases their bioavailability. Look for chelated minerals in supplements.

COENZYME: A nonprotein molecule that binds with a protein molecule in order to form an active enzyme that can then participate in chemical processes.

DAILY VALUE: A term that replaces the RDA (Recommended Dietary Allowance) on food labels. It refers to the percentage of the recommended daily amount of a substance that each serving or dose provides.

DHA (docosahexaenoic acid): A type of omega-3 essential fatty acid found in certain fish.

DIETARY REFERENCE INTAKES (DRIs): A set of values that are the standards for nutrient intake for healthy people in the United States and Canada. The values are based on the average requirements for different sex and age groups and include Estimated Average Requirement (EAR), Recommended Dietary Allowance (RDA), Tolerable Upper Intake Level (UL), and Adequate Intake (AI) values.

EPA (eicosapentaenoic acid): A type of omega-3 essential fatty acid. The body has a limited ability to make EPA by converting alpha-linolenic acid (ALA).

ESSENTIAL FATTY ACIDS: The two fatty acids—linoleic and alpha-linolenic (ALA)—that the body requires but cannot manufacture, which means they must be obtained through diet and/or supplements.

EXTRACTS: The concentrated form of herbs and other natural substances made by treating the natural substance with a solvent and then removing it, leaving the extract behind. Extracts are available as fluids, solids, powders, and tinctures.

FAT-SOLUBLE VITAMINS: Vitamins that can be dissolved in fat and are stored in fat tissue. They include vitamins A, D, E, and K.

FLAVONOIDS: Any of a large group of phytonutrients that are plant pigments; also called bioflavonoids.

FLUID EXTRACT: Herbal extracts that usually have a ratio of one part herb to one part water, alcohol, or both combined.

FREE RADICALS: Unstable molecules that attach themselves to other molecules and damage cells in the process.

NEUROTRANSMITTERS: Chemicals produced by the brain and nerves that transmit and change nerve messages and make it possible for people to feel and think.

PHYTOESTROGENS: These plant chemicals are similar in structure to the hormone estrogen but have a significantly reduced estrogenic effect. Two main types of phytoestrogens are lignans and isoflavones.

PHYTONUTRIENTS: A substance derived from plants, especially one that is neither a vitamin nor mineral, that is beneficial to health.

POLYPHENOLS: Members of a class of phytonutrient found in plants that are potent antioxidants. The word literally means "many phenols," and a phenol is a type of carbon-based molecule.

TINCTURE: A form of herbal supplement in which the herbal extract is mixed in an alcohol base.

WATER-SOLUBLE VITAMINS: Vitamins that are not stored in the body and so must be replaced daily. Examples include the B vitamins and vitamin C.

RESOURCES
Women's Health Resources

Centers for Disease Control and Prevention—Women's Health
www.cdc.gov/women

Dr. Susan Lark—Women's Wellness Today
www.drlark.com

MGH Center for Women's Mental Health
www.womensmentalhealth.org

The National Women's Health Information Center
www.4women.gov
1-800-994-9662

National Women's Health Resource Center
www.healthywomen.org
1-877-986-9472

WebMD—Women's Health
http://women.webmd.com

National Library of Medicine Medline Plus
www.nlm.nih.gov/medlinplus/womenshealth.html

Office of Women's Health
http://www.fda.gov/womens/default.htm

Women's Cancer Information Center
www.womenscancercenter.com

Women's Health Channel
www.womenshealthchannel.com

Women's Health: Where Women Gather, Share and Learn
www.womens-health.com

Women's Heart Association
www.womenheart.org

GENERAL HEALTH, NUTRITION, AND SUPPLEMENT RESOURCES

American Botanical Council
6200 Manor Road
Austin, TX 78723
www.herbalgram.org

Comprehensive information on herbs

Consumer Lab
www.consumerlab.com

Provides independent test results on nutrition products

Dietary Supplements Labels Database
http://dietarysupplements.nlm.nih.gov/dietary

Provides information about the ingredients in more than 2,000 selected brands of dietary supplements, allowing you to compare ingredients in different brands without leaving the house

Food and Nutrition Information Center
http://fnic.nal.usda.gov/nal_display/index.php?info_center=4&tax
_level=1&tax_subject=274

Information on dietary supplements

Health A to Z
www.healthatoz.com

Comprehensive information on consumer health topics

Health Central
www.healthcentral.com

Comprehensive information on consumer health topics

Herb Research Foundation
4140 15th Street
Boulder, CO 80304
www.herbs.org

Comprehensive information on herbs

Linus Pauling Institute
http://lpi.oregonstate.edu/infocenter/

Micronutrient research for optimum health

Mayo Clinic
www.mayoclinic.com

Comprehensive information on consumer health topics

National Center for Complementary and Alternative Medicine
http://nccam.nih.gov/health/supplements.htm

Information on complementary and alternative nutrition and medicine

National Institutes of Health
http://health.nih.gov

Provides information on consumer health topics, clinical trials, research, and more

U.S. Pharmacopeia
www.usp.org

An independent public health organization; offers information on dietary supplements

Wrong Diagnosis
www.wrongdiagnosis.com

Provides information on symptoms, diagnosis, and misdiagnosis of more than 10,000 medical conditions

FOR FURTHER READING

PART I: WOMEN'S MEDICAL AND HEALTH CONCERNS

ACNE

Collier CN et al. The prevalence of acne in adults 20 years and older. *J Am Acad Dermatol* 2008 Jan; 58(1):56–59.

Esler DM et al. The psychosocial experience of women with PCOS—a case control study. *Aust Fam Physician* 2007 Nov; 36(11):965–67.

Seirafi H et al. Assessment of androgens in women with adult-onset acne. *Int J Dermatol* 2007 Nov; 46(11): 1188–91.

Shalita AR et al. Topical nicotinamide compared with clindamycin gel in the treatment of inflammatory acne vulgaris. *Int J Dermatol* 1995; 34:434–37.

Snider B, Dietman DF. Pyridoxine therapy for premenstrual acne flare. *Arch Dermatol* 1974; 110: 130–31.

ADRENAL FATIGUE

Brody S et al. A randomized controlled trial of high dose ascorbic acid for reduction of blood pressure, cortisol, and subjective responses to psychological stress. *Psychopharmacology (Berl)* 2002 Jan; 159(3): 319–24.

Kelly GS. Nutritional and botanical interventions to assist with the adaptation to stress. *Altern Med Rev* 1999 Aug; (4): 249–65.

Monteleone P et al. Effects of phosphatidylserine on the neuroendocrine response to physical stress in humans. *Neuroendocrinology* 1990 Sep; 52(3): 243–48.

Pawlikowski M et al. Effects of six months melatonin treatment on sleep quality and serum concentrations of estradiol, cortisol, dehydroepiandrosterone sulfate, and somatomedin C in elderly women. *Neuroendocrinol Lett* 2002 Apr; 23 Suppl 1:17–19.

Peters EM et al. Vitamin C supplementation attenuates the increases in circulating cortisol, adrenaline and anti-inflammatory polypeptides following ultramarathon running. *Int J Sports Med* 2001 Oct; 22(7): 537–43.

Wilson, James. *Adrenal Fatigue: The 21st Century Syndrome*. Smart Publications, 2002.

AMENORRHEA

Loch EG, Katzorke T. Diagnosis and treatment of dyshormonal menstrual periods in general practice. *Gynakol Praxis* 1990; 149: 489–95.

Milewicz A et al. Vitex agnus castus extract in the treatment of luteal phase defects due to latent hyperprolactinemia. Results of a randomized placebo-controlled double-blind study. *Arzneimittelforschung* 1993; 43:752–56.

Veal L. Complementary therapy and infertility: an Icelandic perspective. *Complement Ther Nurs Midwifery* 1998; 4:3–6.

ANEMIA

Gomez, Joan, MD. *Anemia in Women: Self-Help and Treatment.* Hunter House, 2002.

Iron Disorders Institute. *The Iron Disorders Institute Guide to Anemia.* Cumberland House Publishing, 2003.

ANOREXIA NERVOSA

Birmingham CL, Gritzner S. How does zinc supplementation benefit anorexia nervosa? *Eat Weight Disord* 2006 Dec; 11(4):e109–11.

University of Illinois at Urbana-Champaign (1998, September 8). Data support idea that zinc plays key role in fight against anorexia. *Science Daily.* Retrieved January 22, 2008, from http://www.sciencedaily.com /releases/1998/09/980908073616.htm.

Winston AP et al. Prevalence of thiamin deficiency in anorexia nervosa. *Int J Eat Disord* 2000 Dec; 28(4):451–54.

ANXIETY DISORDERS

Benjamin J et al. Double-blind, placebo-controlled, crossover trial of inositol treatment of panic disorder. *Am J Psychiatry* 1995; 52:1084–86.

Chow YW, Tsang HW. Biopsychosocial effects of qigong as a mindful exercise for people with anxiety disorders: a speculative review. *J Altern Complement Med* 2007 Oct; 13(8): 831–39.

Fux M et al. Inositol treatment of obsessive-compulsive disorder. *Am J Psychiatry* 1996; 153(9): 1219–21.

Geller SE, Studee L. Botanical and dietary supplements for mood and anxiety in menopausal women. *Menopause* 2007 May-Jun; 14(3 Pt 1): 541–49.

Mahady GB. Black cohosh (*Actaea/Cimicifuga race-mosa*): review of the clinical data for safety and efficacy in menopausal symptoms. *Treat Endocrinol* 2005; 4(3): 177–78.

Saeed SA et al. Herbal and dietary supplements for treatment of anxiety disorders. *Am Fam Physician* 2007 Aug 15; 76(4): 549–56.

ASTHMA

Ammon HP. Boswellic acids in chronic inflammatory diseases. *Planta Med* 2006 Oct; 72(12): 1100–16.

Danesch UC. *Petasites hybridus* (Butterbur root) extract in the treatment of asthma—an open trial. *Altern Med Rev* 2004 Mar; 9(1): 54–62.

Gupta I et al. Effects of Boswellia serrata gum resin in patients with bronchial asthma: results of a double-blind, placebo-controlled, 6-week clinical study. *Eur J Med Res* 1998 Nov 17; 3(11): 511–14.

Miyamoto S et al. Fish and fat intake and prevalence of allergic rhinitis in Japanese females: the Osaka Maternal and Child Health Study. *J Am Coll Nutr* 2007 Jun; 26(3): 279–87.

Neuman I et al. Reduction of exercise-induced asthma oxidative stress by lycopene, a natural antioxidant. *Allergy* 2000; 55:1184–89.

Riccioni G et al. Plasma lycopene and antioxidant vitamins in asthma: the PLAVA study. *J Asthma* 2007 Jul-Aug; 44(6): 429–32.

Tecklenburg SL et al. Ascorbic acid supplementation attenuates exercise-induced bronchoconstriction in patients with asthma. *Respir Med* 2007 Aug; 101(8): 1770–78.

BACK PAIN

Mauro GL et al. Vitamin B_{12} in low back pain: a randomized, double-blind, placebo-controlled study. *Eur Rev Med Pharmacol Sci* 2000 May-Jun; 4(3): 53–58.

Vormann J et al. Supplementation with alkaline minerals reduces symptoms in patients with chronic low back pain. *J Trace Elements Med Biol* 2001; 15(2–3): 179–83.

Weiner, Debra K. and Deborah Mitchell. *What Your Doctor May Not Tell You About Back Pain.* Wellness Central, 2007.

BREAST CANCER

Folkers K et al. Enzymology of the response of the carpal tunnel syndrome to riboflavin and to combined riboflavin and pyridoxine. *Proc Natl Acad Sci USA* 1984 Nov; 81(22):7076–78.

Cos S, Sanchez-Barcelo EJ. Melatonin, experimental basis for a possible application in breast cancer prevention and treatment. *Histo Histopath* 2000; 15: 637–47.

Ericson U et al. High folate intake is associated with lower breast cancer incidence in postmenopausal women in the Malmo Diet and Cancer cohort. *Am J Clin Nutr* 2007 Aug; 86(2):434–43.

Farabegoli F et al. (-)-Epigallocatechin-3-gallate down-regulates estrogen receptor alpha function in MCF-7 breast carcinoma cells. *Cancer Detect Prev* 2007 Nov 29.

Schernhammer E, Hankinson S. Urinary melatonin levels and breast cancer risk. *J Nat Can Instit* 2005; 97(14): 1084–87.

Thangapazham RL et al. Green tea polyphenol and epi-gallocatechin gallate induce apoptosis and inhibit invasion in human breast cancer cells. *Cancer Biol Ther* 2007 Sep 1;6(12).

Wu AH, et al. Green tea and risk of breast cancer in Asian Americans. *Intl J Cancer* 2003; 106(Sept. 10):574–79.

CERVICAL CANCER
Hernandez BY et al. Diet and premalignant lesions of the cervix: evidence of a protective role for folate, fiboflain, thiamin, and vitamin B_{12}. *Cancer Causes Control* 2003 Nov; 14(9): 859–70.

Keane, Maureen and Daniella Chace. *What to Eat if You Have Cancer.* McGraw-Hill, 2006.

Nagata C et al. Serum carotenoids and vitamins and risk of cervical dysplasia from a case-control study in Japan. *Br J Cancer* 1999 Dec; 81(7): 1234–37.

Palan PR et al. Beta-carotene levels in exfoliated cervicovaginal epithelial cells in cervical intraepithelial neoplasia and cervical cancer. *Am J Obstet Gynecol* 1992 Dec; 167(6): 1899–1903.

Szarawski, Anne. *Preventing Cervical Cancer: What Every Woman Should Know.* Altman Publishing, 2007.

CHLAMYDIA
Breguet, Amy. *Chlamydia.* Rosen Publishing Group, 2006.

Meyers DS et al. Screening for chlamydial infection: an evidence update for the U.S. Preventive Services Task Force. *Ann Intern Med* 2007 Jul 17; 147(2): 135–42.

CHRONIC FATIGUE SYNDROME

Bentler SE et al. Prospective observational study of treatments for unexplained chronic fatigue. *J Clin Psychiatry* 2005 May; 66(5): 625–32.

Hartz AJ et al. Randomized controlled trial of Siberian ginseng for chronic fatigue. *Psychol Med* 2004 Jan; 3491): 51–61.

Heap LC et al. Vitamin B status in patients with chronic fatigue syndrome. *J R Soc Med* 1999 Apr; 92(4): 183–85.

Maes M et al. Lower serum zinc in chronic fatigue syndrome (CFS): relationships to immune dysfunctions and relevance for the oxidative stress status in CFS. *J Affect Disord* 2006 Feb; 90(2–3): 141–47.

Puri BK. The use of eicosapentaenoic acid in the treatment of chronic fatigue syndrome. *Prostaglandins Leukot Essent Fatty Acids* 2004 Apr; 70(4): 399–401.

Rai D et al. Anti-stress effects of *Ginkgo biloba* and *Panax ginseng*: a comparative study. *J Pharmacol Sci* 2003 Dec; 93(4): 458–64.

CONSTIPATION

Berkson, D. Lindsey. *Healthy Digestion the Natural Way: Preventing and Healing Heartburn, Constipation, Gas, Diarrhea, Inflammatory Bowel and Gallbladder Diseases, Ulcers, Irritable Bowel Syndrome, and More.* Wiley, 2000.

Odes HS, Madar Z. A double-blind trial of a celandine, aloe vera and psyllium laxative preparation in adult patients with constipation. *Digestion* 1991; 49(2): 65–71.

Trepel F. Dietary fibre: more than a matter of dietetics. II. Preventative and therapeutic uses. *Wien Klin Wochenschr* 2004 Aug 31; 116(15–16): 511–22.

DEPRESSION

Astorg P et al. Association of folate intake with the occurrence of depressive episodes in middle-aged French men and women. *Br J Nutr* 2007 Dec 6;1–5.

Delle CR et al. Efficacy and tolerability of oral and intramuscular S-adenosyl-L-methionine 1,4-butanedisulfonate (SAMe) in the treatment of major depression: comparison with imipramine in 2 multicenter studies. *Am J Clin Nutr*. 2002 Nov; 76(5):1172S–6S.

Geller SE, Studee L. Botanical and dietary supplements for mood and anxiety in menopausal women. *Menopause*. 2007 May-Jun; 14(3 Pt 1):541–49.

Mischoulon D, Raab MF. The role of folate in depression and dementia. *J Clin Psychiatry* 2007; 68 Suppl 10:28–33.

Pancheri P et al. A double-blind, randomized parallel-group, efficacy and safety study of intramuscular S-adenosyl-L-methionine 1,4-butanedisulphonate (SAMe) versus imipramine in patients with major depressive disorder. *Int J Neuropsychopharmacol* 2002 Dec; 5(4):287–94.

Poldinger W et al. A functional-dimensional approach to depression: serotonin deficiency as a target syndrome in a comparison of 5-hydroxytryptophan and fluvoxamine. *Psychopathology* 24:53–81, 1991.

Schachter, Michael B, MD. *What Your Doctor May Not Tell You About Depression.* St. Martin's, 2006.

DIABETES

Anderson RA. Chromium and polyphenols from cinnamon improve insulin sensitivity. *Proc Nutr Soc* 2008 Feb; 67(1):48–53.

Hummel M et al. Chromium in metabolic and cardiovascular disease. *Horm Metab Res* 2007 Oct; 39(10): 743–51.

Joyal, Steven, MD. *What Your Doctor May* Not *Tell You About Diabetes.* St. Martin's, 2007.

Pittas AG et al. Vitamin D and calcium intake in relation to type 2 diabetes in women. *Diabetes Care.* 2006 Mar; 29(3):650–56.

Sharma A et al. Serum magnesium: an early predictor of course and complications of diabetes mellitus. *J Indian Med Assoc* 2007 Jan; 105(1):16, 18, 20.

DRY EYE SYNDROME

Chainani W. Safety and anti-inflammatory activity of curcumin: a component of turmeric (*Curcuma longa*). *Altern Complement Med* 2003; 9:161–68.

Kobayashi TK et al. Effect of retinol palmitate as a treatment for dry eye: a cytological evaluation. *Opthalmologica* 1997; 211(6): 358–61.

Miljanovic B et al. Relation between dietary n-3 and n-6 fatty acids and clinically diagnosed dry eye syndrome in women. *Am J Clin Nutr* 2005 Oct; 82(4):887–93.

Pinheiro MN Jr et al. [Oral flaxseed oil (Linum usitatissimum) in the treatment for dry-eye Sjögren's syndrome patients]. *Arg Bras Oftalmol* 2007 Jul-Aug; 70(4):649–55.

Schaumberg DA et al. Prevalence of dry eye syndrome among US women. *Am J Ophthalmol* 2003 Aug; 136(2):318–26.

ENDOMETRIAL CANCER
Hirsch K et al. Effect of purified allicin, the major ingredient of freshly crushed garlic, on cancer cell proliferation. *Nutr Cancer* 2000; 39(2): 245–54.

Horn-Ross PL et al. Phytoestrogen intake and endometrial cancer risk. *J Natl Cancer Inst* 2003 Aug 6; 95(15):1158–64.

Worwood, Valerie Ann and Julia Stonehouse. *The Endometriosis Natural Treatment Program: A Complete Self-Help Plan for Improving Health and Well-Being.* New World Library, 2007.

Ziaei S et al. A randomized, controlled trial of vitamin E in the treatment of primary dysmenorrhoea. *BJOG* 2005; 112(4): 466–69.

Ziaei S et al. A randomized, placebo-controlled trial to determine the effect of vitamin E in treatment of primary dysmenorrheal. *BJOG* 2001; 108:1181–83.

FIBROCYSTIC BREAST CHANGES
Boyle CA et al. Caffeine consumption and fibrocystic breast disease: a case-control epidemiologic study. *J Natl Cancer Inst* 1984; 72(5): 1015–19.

Low Dog T. Integrative treatments for premenstrual syndrome. *Alt Ther Health Med* 2001; 7(5): 32–39.

Girman A et al. An integrative medicine approach to premenstrual syndrome. *Am J Obstet Gynec* 2003; 188(5 Suppl): S56–S65.

Horner NK, Lampe JW. Potential mechanisms of diet therapy for fibrocystic breast conditions show inadequate evidence of effectiveness. *J Am Diet Assoc* 2000 Nov; 100(11): 1368–80.

FIBROMYALGIA

Caruso I et al. Double-blind study of 5-hydroxytryptophan versus placebo in the treatment of primary fibromyalgia syndrome. *J Int Med Res* 1990; 18:201–9.

Jacobsen S et al. Oral S-adenosylmethionine in primary fibromyalgia. Double-blind clinical evaluation. *Scand J Rheumatol* 1991; 20(4): 294–302.

Lister RE. An open, pilot study to evaluate the potential benefits of coenzyme Q_{10} combined with *Ginkgo biloba* extract in fibromyalgia syndrome. *J Int Med Res* 2002 Mar-Apr; 30(2):195–99.

St. Amand, R. Paul and Claudia Craig Marek. *What Your Doctor May Not Tell You About Fibromyalgia.* Wellness Central, 2006.

Tavoni A et al. Evaluation of S-adenosylmethionine in primary fibromyalgia. A double-blind crossover study. *Am J Med* 1987; 83(5A): 107–10.

Volkmann H et al. Double-blind, placebo-controlled cross-over study of intravenous S-adenosyl-L-methionine in patients with fibromyalgia. *Scand J Rheumatol* 1997; 26(3): 206–11.

GALLSTONES

Cuevas A et al. Diet as a risk factor for cholesterol gallstone disease. *J Am Coll Nutr* 2004 Jun; 23(3):187–96.

Hussain MS, Chandrasekhara N. Effect of curcumin on cholesterol gallstone induction in mice. *Indian J Med Res* 1992 Oct; 96:288–91.

Simon JA, Hudes ES. Serum ascorbic acid and other correlates of gallbladder disease among US adults. *Am J Public Health* 1998 Aug; 88(8):1208–12.

HAIR LOSS
Deloche C et al. Low iron stores: a risk factor for excessive hair loss in non-menopausal women. *Eur J Dermatol* 2007 Nov-Dec; 17(6):507–12.

Trost LB et al. The diagnosis and treatment of iron deficiency and its potential relationship to hair loss. *J Am Acad Dermatol* 2006 May; 54(5):824–44.

HEADACHE/MIGRAINE
Birdsall TC. 5-Hydroxytryptophan: a clinically-effective serotonin precursor. *Alt Med Review* 1998; 3(4):271–80.

Diener HC et al. The first placebo-controlled trial of a special butterbur root extract for the prevention of migraine: reanalysis of efficacy criteria. *Eur Neurol* 2004; 51(2):89–97.

Diener HC et al. Efficacy and safety of 6.25 mg t.i.d. feverfew CO_2-extract (MIG-99) in migraine prevention—a randomized, double-blind, multicentre, placebo-controlled study. *Cephalalgia* 2005; 25(11):1031–41.

Dzugan, Sergey, MD. *The Migraine Cure.* Dragon Door Publishers, 2006.

Ernst E, Pittler MH. The efficacy and safety of feverfew (*Tanacetum parthenium* L.): an update of a systematic review. *Public Health Nutr* 2000; 3(4A): 509–14.

Evans RW, Taylor FR. "Natural" or alternative medications for migraine prevention. *Headache* 2006; 46(6): 1012–18.

Gatto G et al. Analgesizing effect of a methyl donor (S-adenosylmethionine) in migraine: an open clinical trial. *Int J Clin Pharmacol Res* 1986; 6:15–17.

Hershey AD et al. Coenzyme Q_{10} deficiency and response to supplementation in pediatric and adolescent migraine. *Headache* 2007 Jan; 47(1):73–80.

Lipton RB et al. Petasites hybridus root (butterbur) is an effective preventive treatment for migraine. *Neurology* 2004 Dec 28; 63(12): 2240–44.

Mauskop A, Altura BM. Role of magnesium in the pathogenesis and treatment of migraines. *Clin Neurosci* 1998; 5(1):24–27.

Sandor PS et al. Efficacy of coenzyme Q_{10} in migraine prophylaxis: a randomized controlled trial. *Neurology* 2005 Feb 22; 64(4):713–15.

HEART DISEASE

Bazzano LA et al. Effect of folic acid supplementation on risk of cardiovascular diseases: a meta-analysis of randomized controlled trials. *JAMA* 2006 Dec 13; 296(22):2720–26.

Clarke E et al. Effects of B-vitamins on plasma homocysteine concentrations and on risk of cardiovascular disease and dementia. *Curr Opin Clin Nutr Metab Care* 2007 Jan; 10(1):32–39.

Goldberg, Nieca MD. *The Women's Healthy Heart Program: Lifesaving Strategies for Preventing and Healing Heart Disease.* Ballantine, 2006.

Malik S, Kashyap ML. Niacin, lipids, and heart disease. *Curr Cardiol Rep* 2003 Nov; 5(6):470–76.

Pepe S et al. Coenzyme Q_{10} in cardiovascular disease. *Mitochondrion* 2007 Jun; 7 Suppl:S154–67.

Sesso H et al. Dietary lycopene, tomato-based food products, and cardiovascular disease in women. *J Nutr* 2003; 133(7):2336–41.

Stevinson C et al. Garlic for treating hypercholesterolemia. A meta-analysis of randomized clinical trials. *Ann Intern Med* 2000; 133:420–29.

Yu BL, Zhao SP. Anti-inflammatory effect is an important property of niacin on atherosclerosis beyond its lipid-altering effects. *Med Hypotheses* 2007; 69(1):90–94.

HEMORRHOIDS

Abramowitz L et al. Anal fissure and thrombosed external hemorrhoids before and after delivery. *Dis Colon Rectum* 2002; 45:650–55.

Alonso-Coelle P et al. Fiber for the treatment of hemorrhoids complications: a systematic review and meta-analysis. *Am J Gastroenterol* 2006 Jan; 101(1):181–88.

Perez-Miranda M et al. Effect of fiber supplements on internal bleeding hemorrhoids. *Hepatogastroenterology* 1996 Nov-Dec; 43(12):1504–47.

Sirtori CR. Aescin: pharmacology, pharmacokinetics and therapeutic profile. *Pharmacol Res* 2001 Sep; 44(3):183–93.

Wald A. Constipation, diarrhea, and symptomatic hemorrhoids during pregnancy. *Gastroenterol Clin North Am* 2003; 32:309–22, vii.

HERPES

Brown ZA et al. Genital herpes complicating pregnancy. *Obstet Gynecol* 2005 Oct; 106(4):845–56.

Ebel, Charles. *Managing Herpes: Living and Loving with HSV.* American Social Health Association, 2007.

Femiano F et al. Recurrent herpes labialis: a pilot study of the efficacy of zinc therapy. *J Oral Pathol Med* 2005 Aug; 34(7):423–25.

www.herpes.org—Neonatal Herpes University of Washington Academic Medical Center, Children's Hospital and Regional Medical Center, 1998.

HIGH BLOOD PRESSURE (HYPERTENSION)

American Heart Association, http://www.americanheart.org/presenter.jhtml?identifier=2123.

Dhawan V, Jain S. Garlic supplementation prevents oxidative DNA damage in essential hypertension. *Mol Cell Biochem* 2005 Jul; 275(1–2):85–94.

Militante JD, Lombardini JB. Treatment of hypertension with oral taurine: experimental and clinical studies. *Amino Acids* 2002; 23(4):381–93;

Podymow T, August P. Hypertension in pregnancy. *Adv Chronic Kidney Dis* 2007 Apr; 14(2):178–90.

Rahman K, Lowe GM. Garlic and cardiovascular disease: a critical review. *J Nutr* 2006 Mar; 136(3 Suppl):736S–740S.

Walker AF et al. Hypotensive effects of hawthorn for patients with diabetes taking prescription drugs: a randomised controlled trial. *Br J Gen Pract* 2006 Jun; 56(527):437–43.

Wang L et al. Dietary intake of dairy products, calcium, and vitamin D and the risk of hypertension in middle-aged and older women. *Hypertension* 2008 Feb 7.

Yoshioka M et al. Central hypotensive effect involving neurotransmitters of long-term administration of taurine to stroke-prone spontaneously hypertensive rat. *Masui* 2007 Feb; 56(2):139–47.

HYPOTHYROIDISM
Menif O et al. Hypothyroidism and pregnancy: impact on mother and child health. *Ann Biol Clin (Paris)* 2008 Jan 29;66(1):43–51.

Shomon, Mary J. *Living Well with Hypothyroidism: What Your Doctor Doesn't Tell You . . . That You Need To Know.* Collins, 2005.

INCONTINENCE
Elkins, Rita. *Natural Treatment for Urinary Incontinence: Using Butterbur and Other Natural Supplements to Treat Bladder-Control Problems.* Woodland Health, 2000.

Kegel exercises information provided by the National Institute of Diabetes and Digestive and Kidney Diseases: http://kidney.niddk.nih.gov/kudiseases/pubs/exercise_ez/

Petasites hybridus. *Altern Med Rev* 2001 Apr; 6(2): 207–9.

INFERTILITY
Czeizel AE et al. The effect of preconceptional multivita-min supplementation on fertility. *Internat J Vit Nutr Res* 1996; 66:55–58.

Lukse MP, Vacc NA. Grief, depression, and coping in women undergoing infertility treatment. *Obstet and Gynecol* 1999; 93(2): 245–51.

Nachtigall RD et al. The effects of gender-specific diagnosis on men's and women's response to infertility. *Fertil Steril* 1992 Jan;57(1):113–21.

Westphal LM et al. Double-blind, placebo-controlled study of Fertilityblend: a nutritional supplement for improving fertility in women. *Clin Exp Obstet Gynecol* 2006; 33(4):205–8.

INSOMNIA
Murray, Michael ND. *5-HTP: The Natural Way to Overcome Depression, Obesity, and Insomnia.* Bantam, 1999.

Williamson, Karen. *Sleep Deep (52 Brilliant Ways).* Perigee Trade, 2007.

IRRITABLE BOWEL SYNDROME
Camilleri M. Probiotics and irritable bowel syndrome: Rationale, putative mechanisms, and evidence of clinical efficacy. *J Clin Gastroenterol* 2006 Mar; 40(3):264–69.

Hale LP. Proteolytic activity and immunogenicity of oral bromelain within the gastrointestinal tract of mice. *Int Immunopharmacol* 2004 Feb; 4(2):255–64.

Langmead L, Rampton DS. Review article: Herbal treatment in gastrointestinal and liver disease—benefits and dangers. *Aliment Pharmacol Ther* 2001 Sep; 15(9):1239–52.

Tomas-Ridocci M et al. The efficacy of *Plantago ovata* as a regulator of intestinal transit. A double-blind study compared to placebo. *Rev Esp Enferm Dig* 1992 Jul; 82(1):17–22.

Wangen, Stephen, MD. *The Irritable Bowel Syndrome Solution: How It's Cured at the IBS Treatment Center.* Innate Health Publishing, 2006.

LUPUS

Crosbie D et al. Dehydroepiandrosterone for systemic lupus erythematosus. *Cochrane Database Syst Rev*. 2007 Oct 17; (4):CD005114.

Digeronimo, Theresa Foy and Sara J. Henry. *New Hope for People with Lupus*. Three Rivers Press, 2002.

Nordmark G et al. Effects of dehydroepiandrosterone supplement on health-related quality of life in gluco-corticoid treated female patients with systemic lupus erythematosus. *Autoimmunity* 2005 Nov; 38(7):531–40.

Pigache, Philippa. *Positive Options for Living with Lupus: Self-Help and Treatment*. Hunter House, 2006.

Wright SA et al. A randomised placebo-controlled interventional trial of omega-3-polyunsaturated fatty acids on endothelial function and disease activity in systemic lupus erythematosus. *Ann Rheum Dis* 2007 Sep 17.

MENOPAUSE

Coon JT et al. Trifolium pratense isoflavones in the treatment of menopausal hot flushes: a systematic review and meta-analysis. *Phytomedicine* 2007 Feb;14(2–3):153–59.

Northrup, Christiane, MD. *The Wisdom of Menopause: Creating Physical and Emotional Health and Healing During the Change,* 2nd ed. Bantam, 2006.

Oktem M et al. Black cohosh and fluoxetine in the treatment of postmenopausal symptoms: a prospective, randomized trial. *Adv Ther* 2007 Mar-Apr; 24(2):448–61.

Pruthi S et al. Pilot evaluation of flaxseed for the management of hot flashes. *J Soc Integr Oncol* 2007 Summer; 5(3):106–12.

Rotem C, Kaplan B. Phyto-Female Complex for the relief of hot flushes, night sweats and quality of sleep: randomized, controlled, double-blind pilot study. *Gynecol Endocrinol* 2007 Feb; 23(2):117–22.

MORNING SICKNESS

Erick, Miriam. *Managing Morning Sickness: A Survival Guide for Pregnant Women.* Bull Publishing, 2004.

Niebyl JR, Goodwin TM. Overview of nausea and vomiting of pregnancy with an emphasis on vitamins and ginger. *Am J Obstet Gynecol* 2002; 186:S253–S255.

OBESITY AND OVERWEIGHT

Birdsall TC. 5-hydroxytryptophan: a clinically-effective serotonin precursor. *Alt Med Rev* 1998; 3(4): 271–80.

Blaak E. Gender differences in fat metabolism. *Curr Opin Clin Nutr Metab Care* 2001 Nov; 4(6):499–502.

Boschmann M, Thielecke F. The effects of epigallo-catechin-3-gallate on thermogenesis and fat oxidation in obese men: a pilot study. *J Am Coll Nutr* 2007 Aug; 26(4):389S–395S.

Hellstrom L et al. Mechanisms behind gender differences in circulating leptin levels. *J Intern Med* 2000; 247(4): 457–62.

Lin JK, Lin-Shiau SY. Mechanisms of hypolipidemic and anti-obesity effects of tea and tea polyphenols. *Mol Nutr Food Res* 2006 Feb; 50(2):211–17.

Lovejoy JC. The influence of sex hormones on obesity across the female life span. *J Womens Health* 1998; 7(10):1247–56.

Wilsgaard T et al. Impact of body weight on blood pressure with a focus on sex differences: the Tromso Study, 1986–1995. *Arch Intern Med* 2000; 160(18): 2847–53.

OSTEOARTHRITIS

Bales, Peter. *Osteoarthritis: Preventing and Healing Without Drugs.* Prometheus Books, 2008.

Bradley JD et al. A randomized, double blind, placebo controlled trial of intravenous loading with S-adenosylmethionine (SAM) followed by oral SAM therapy in patients with knee osteoarthritis. *J Rheumatol* 1994; 21(5): 905–11.

Gregory PJ et al. Dietary supplements for osteoarthritis. *Am Fam Physician* 2008 Jan 15; 77(2):177–84.

Kim LS et al. Efficacy of methylsulfonylmethane (MSM) in osteoarthritis pain of the knee: a pilot clinical trial. *Osteoarthritis Cartilage* 2006 Mar; 14(3): 286–94.

McCleane G et al. The analgesic efficacy of topical capsaicin is enhanced by glyceryl trinitrate in painful osteoarthritis: a randomized, double blind, placebo controlled study. *Eur J Pain* 2000;4(4): 355–60.

Mehta K et al. Comparison of glucosamine sulfate and a polyherbal supplement for the relief of osteoarthritis of the knee: a randomized controlled trial. *BMC Complement Altern Med* 2007 Oct 31; 7:34.

Newnham RE. Essentiality of boron for healthy bones and joints. *Environ Health Perspect* 1994 Nov; 102 Suppl 7:83–85.

Shakibaei M et al. Suppression of NF-kappaB activation by curcumin leads to inhibition of expression of cyclo-oxygenase-2 and matrix metalloproteinase-9 in human articular chondrocytes: implications for the treatment of osteoarthritis. *Biochem Pharmacol* 2007 May 1; 73(9):1434–45.

OSTEOPOROSIS

Arjmandi BH. The role of phytoestrogens in the prevention and treatment of osteoporosis in ovarian hormone deficiency. *J Am Coll Nutr* 2001 Oct; 20(5 Suppl): 398S–402S.

Atkinson C et al. The effects of phytoestrogen isoflavones on bone density in women: a double-blind, randomized,plaebo-controlled trial. *Am J Clin Nutr* 2004; 79:326–33.

Nelson, Miriam E., MD. *Strong Women, Strong Bones: Everything You Need to Know to Prevent, Treat and Beat Osteoporosis.* Perigee Trade, 2001.

Song WO et al. Soy isoflavones as safe functional ingredients. *J Med Food* 2007 Dec; 10(4): 571–80.

Ye YB et al. Soy isoflavones attenuate bone loss in early postmenopausal Chinese women: a single-blind randomized, placebo-controlled trial. *Eur J Nutr* 2006 Jun 8.

OVARIAN CANCER

Dizon, Don S, MD. *100 Questions and Answers About Ovarian Cancer,* 2nd ed. Jones & Bartlett, 2006.

Goff BA et al. Frequency of symptoms of ovarian cancer in women presenting to primary care clinics. *JAMA* 2004; 291:2705–12.

Kowalska E et al. Increased rates of chromosome breakage in BRCA1 carriers are normalized by oral selenium supplementation. *Cancer Epidemiol Biomarkers Prev* 2005 May; 14(5):1302–6.

Ye B et al. *Ginkgo biloba* and ovarian cancer prevention: epidemiological and biological evidence. *Cancer Lett* 2007 Jun 18; 251(1):43–52.

Zhang M et al. Intake of specific carotenoids and the risk of epithelial ovarian cancer. *Br J Nutr* 2007 Jul; 98(1):187–93.

PELVIC INFLAMMATORY DISEASE

Cabrera C et al. Beneficial effects of green tea—a review. *J Am Coll Nutr* 2006; 25(2):79–99.

Das M et al. Inhibition of tumor growth and inflammation by consumption of tea. *Phytother Res* 2002; 16 (Suppl 1):S40–44.

Hillis SD et al. Delayed care of pelvic inflammatory disease as a risk factor for impaired fertility. *Am J Obstet Gynecol* 1993 May; 168(5):1503–9.

O'Donnell, Judith A. *Pelvic Inflammatory Disease.* Chelsea House Publications, 2006.

PREMENSTRUAL SYNDROME (PMS)

Bertone-Johnson ER et al. Calcium and vitamin D intake and risk of incident premenstrual syndrome. *Arch Intern Med* 2005 Jun 13; 165(11):1246–52.

Jones, Andrew, MD. *The All-Natural Cure to Your PMS.* 48 Hour Books, 2007.

Lee, John, Jesse Hanley and Virginia Hopkins. *What Your Doctor May* Not *Tell You About Premenopause.* Grand Central, 2005.

Quaranta S et al. Pilot study of the efficacy and safety of a modified-release magnesium 250 mg tablet (Sincromag) for the treatment of premenstrual syndrome. *Clin Drug Investig* 2007; 27(1):51–58.

Schellenberg R. Treatment for the premenstrual syndrome with agnus castus fruit extract: prospective, randomized, placebo-controlled study. *BJM* 2001; 20;134–37.

Wuttke W et al. Chaste tree (*Vitex agnus-castus*)— pharmacology and clinical indications. *Phytomedicine* 2003 May; 10(4):348–57.

RHEUMATOID ARTHRITIS

Ammon HP. Boswellic acids in chronic inflammatory diseases. *Planta Med* 2006 Oct; 72(12):1100–16.

Fischer, Harry D, MD and Winnie Yu. *What to Do When the Doctor Says It's Rheumatoid Arthritis.* Fair Winds Press, 2005.

Funk JL et al. Turmeric extracts containing curcuminoids prevent experimental rheumatoid arthritis. *J Nat Prod* 2006 Mar; 69(3):351–55.

Goldberg RJ, Katz J. A meta-analysis of the analgesic effects of omega-3 polyunsaturated fatty acid supplementation for inflammatory joint pain. *Pain* 2007 May; 129(1–2):210–23.

Karlson EW et al. Do breast-feeding and other reproductive factors influence future risk of

rheumatoid arthritis? *Arthritis Rheum* 2004 Nov;
50(11):3458–67.

Park C et al. Curcumin induces apoptosis and inhibits
prostaglandin E(2) production in synovial fibroblasts of
patients with rheumatoid arthritis. *Int J Mol Med* 2007
Sep; 20(3):365–72.

Ryan-Harshman J, Aldoori W. The relevance of selenium
to immunity, cancer, and infectious/inflammatory
diseases. *Can J Diet Pract Res* 2005 Summer; 66(2):
98–102.

Yazar M et al. Synovial fluid and plasma selenium,
copper, zinc, and iron concentrations in patients with
rheumatoid arthritis and osteoarthritis. *Biol Trace Elem
Res* 2005 Aug; 106(2):123–32.

SCLERODERMA
Herrick Al et al. Micronutrient antioxidant status in
patients with primary Raynaud's phenomenon and
systemic sclerosis. *J Rheumatol* 1994 Aug;21(8):
1477–83.

Mayes, Maureen D, MD. *The Scleroderma Book: A Guide
for Patients and Families.* Oxford University Press,
2005.

SHINGLES
Siegel, Mary-Ellen. *Living with Shingles: New Hope for
an Old Disease.* M. Evans, 2002.

Walsh DE et al. Subjective response to lysine in the
therapy of herpes simplex. *J Antimicrob Chemother* 1983
Nov; 12(5):489–96.

TEMPOROMANDIBULAR JOINT SYNDROME

LeResche L et al. Use of exogenous hormones and risk of temporomandibular disorder pain. *Pain* 1997 Jan; 69(1–2): 153–60.

Uppgaard, Robert O. *Taking Control of TMJ: Your Total Wellness Program for Recovering from Temporomandibular Joint Pain, Whiplash, Fibromyalgia, and Related Disorders.* New Harbinger, 1999.

URINARY TRACT INFECTION

Foxman B et al. Urinary tract infection: self-reported incidence and associated costs. *Ann Epidemiol* 2000; 10:509–15.

Kilmartin, Angela. *The Patient's Encyclopedia of Urinary Tract Infection, Sexual Cystitis and Interstitial Cystitis.* New Century Press, 2004.

Stothers L. A randomized trial to evaluate effectiveness and cost effectiveness of naturopathic cranberry products as prophylaxis against urinary tract infection in women. *Can J Urol* 2002; 9:1558–62.

Walker EB et al. Cranberry concentrate: UTI prophylaxis. *J Fam Pract* 1997; 45:167–68.

VAGINITIS

Delia A et al. Effectiveness of oral administration of Lactobacillus paracasei subsp. paracasei F19 in association with vaginal suppositories of Lactobacillus acidofilus in the treatment of vaginosis and in the prevention of recurrent vaginitis. *Minerva Ginecol* 2006 Jun; 58(3):227–31.

Falagas ME et al. Probiotics for the treatment of women with bacterial vaginosis. *Clin Microbiol Infect* 2007 Jul; 13(7):657–64.

Koch, Heinrich P. *Garlic: The Science and Therapeutic Application of Allium Savivum and Related Species.* Williams & Wilkins, 1996.

Mondello F. In vivo activity of terpinen-4-ol, the main bioactive component of *Melaleuca alternifolia* Cheel (tea tree) oil against azole-susceptible and -resistant human pathogenic Candida species. *BMC Infect Dis* 2006 Nov 3; 6:158.

Wilson C. Recurrent vulvovaginitis candidiasis; an overview of traditional and alternative therapies. *Adv Nurse Pract* 2005 May; 13(5):24–29.

VARICOSE VEINS

Bielanski TE, Piotrowski ZH: Horse-chestnut seed extract for chronic venous insufficiency. *J Fam Pract* 1999; 48:171–72.

Dattner AM. From medical herbalism to phytotherapy in dermatology: back to the future. *Dermatol Ther* 2003; 16(2):106–13.

Pittler MH, Ernst E. Horse-chestnut seed extract for chronic venous insufficiency: a criteria-based systemic review. *Arch Dermatol* 1998; 134;1356–60.

Rathbun SW, Kirkpatrick AC. Treatment of chronic venous insufficiency. *Curr Treat Options Cardiovasc Med* 2007 Apr; 9(2):115–26.

Suter A. Treatment of patients with venous insufficiency with fresh plant horse chestnut seed extract: a review of 5 clinical studies. *Adv Ther* 2006 Jan-Feb;23(1):179–90.

PART II: SUPPLEMENTS
Vitamins and Minerals

B VITAMINS
Gerli S et al. Effects of inositol on ovarian function and metabolic factors in women with PCOS: a randomized double-blind placebo-controlled trial. *Eur Rev Med Pharmacol Sci* 2003 Nov-Dec; 7(6):151–59.

VITAMIN A
Russell RM. The vitamin A spectrum: from deficiency to toxicity. *Am J Clin Nutr* 2000; 71(4):878–84.

Zhang S et al. Dietary carotenoids and vitamins A, C, and E and risk of breast cancer. *J Natl Cancer Inst* 1999; 91(6):547–56.

VITAMIN C
Morton DJ. Vitamin C supplement use and bone mineral density in postmenopausal women. *J Bone Min Res* 2001; 16:135–40.

Simon JA, Hudes ES. Serum ascorbic acid and gallbladder disease prevalence among US adults: the Third National Health and Nutrition Examination Survey (NHANES III). *Arch Intern Med* 2000 Apr 10; 160(7):931–36.

VITAMIN D
Dawson-Hughes B, Bischoff-Ferrari HA. Therapy of osteoporosis with calcium and vitamin D. *J Bone Miner Res* 2007 Dec; 22 Suppl. 2:V59–63

Garland CF et al. The role of vitamin D in cancer prevention. *Am J Public Health* 2006 Feb; 96(2):252–61.

Holick, Michael D., MD and Mark Jenkins. *The UV Advantage*. IBook, 2007.

VITAMIN E
U.S. Dept. of Agriculture, Agricultural Research Service
2004; USDA National Nutrient Database for Standard
Reference, Release 16–1, http://www.ars.usda.gov/ba/
bhnrc/ndl.

Various authors and articles regarding the Women's
Health Study in *JAMA,* July 6, 2005; vol. 294.

VITAMIN K
Feskanich D et al. Vitamin K intake and hip fractures in
women: a prospective study. *Am J Clin Nutr* 1999 Jan;
69(1):74–79.

Francucci CM et al. Role of vitamin K on biochemical
markers, bone mineral density, and fracture risk.
J Endocrinol Invest 2007; 30(6 Suppl):24–28.

Pearson DA. Bone health and osteoporosis: the role of
vitamin K and potential antagonism by anticoagulants.
Nutr Clin Pract 2007 Oct; 22(5):517–44.

BORON
Hunt CD et al. Metabolic responses of postmenopausal
women to supplemental dietary boron and aluminum
during usual and low magnesium intake: boron, calcium,
and magnesium absorption and retention and blood
mineral concentrations. *Am J Clin Nutr* 1997 Mar;
65(3):803–13.

CALCIUM
Fuchs, Nan Kathryn. *User's Guide to Calcium and
Magnesium.* Basic Health, 2002.

Rizzoli R et al. The role of calcium and vitamin D in the
management of osteoporosis. *Bone* 2008 Feb;
42(2):246–49.

Schaafsma A et al. Delay of natural bone loss by higher intakes of specific minerals and vitamins. *Crit Rev Food Sci Nutr* 2001 May; 41(4):225–49.

CHROMIUM

Hummel M et al. Chromium in metabolic and cardiovascular disease. *Horm Metab Res* 2007 Oct; 39(10):743–51.

Smith, Melissa Dane. *User's Guide to Chromium.* Basic Health, 2002.

COPPER

Crayton JW, Walsh WJ. Elevated serum copper levels in women with a history of post-partum depression. *J Trace Elem Med Biol* 2007; 21(1):17–21.

Trumbo P et al. Food and Nutrition Board, Institute of Medicine, the National Academies. Dietary reference intakes: vitamin A, vitamin K, arsenic, boron, chromium, copper, iodine, iron, manganese, molybdenum, nickel, silicon, vanadium, and zinc. *J Am Diet Assoc* 2001 Mar; 101(3):294–301.

IRON

Gomez, Jean, MD. *Anemia in Women: Self-Help and Treatment.* Hunter House, 2002.

Davidsson L. Approaches to improve iron bioavailability from complemenary foods. *J Nutr* 2003; 133:1560S–2S.

MAGNESIUM

Ascherio A et al. A prospective study of nutritional factors and hypertension among US men. *Circulation* 1992; 86(5):1475–84.

Bianchi A et al. Role of magnesium, coenzyme Q_{10}, riboflavin, and vitamin B_{12} in migraine prophylaxis. *Vitam Horm* 2004; 69:297–312.

Peikert A et al. Prophylaxis of migraine with oral magnesium: results from a prospective, multi-center, placebo-controlled and double-blind randomized study. *Cephalalgia* 1996 Jun; 16(4):257–63.

MANGANESE
Bendich A. The potential for dietary supplements to reduce premenstrual syndrome (PMS) symptoms. *J Am Coll Nutr* 2000; 19(1):3–11.

Okano T. Effects of essential trace elements on bone turnover—in relation to osteoporosis. *Nippon Rinsho* 1996 Jan; (491):148–54.

PHOSPHORUS
Heaney RP. Phosphorus nutrition and the treatment of osteoporosis. *Mayo Clin Proc* 2004; 79:91–97.

Kemi VE et al. High phosphorus intakes acutely and negatively affect Ca and bone metabolism in a dose-dependent manner in healthy young females. *Br J Nutr* 2006 Sept; 96(3):545–52.

POTASSIUM
Institute of Medicine report, November 2004: Dietary Reference Intakes: Water, Potassium, Sodium, Chloride, and Sulfate, http://www.iom.edu/?id=18495&redirect=0.

SELENIUM
Kadrobova J et al. Selenium status is decreased in patients with intrinsic asthma. *Biol Trace Elem Res* 1996; 52:241–48.

Turan B et al. Selenium combined with vitamin E and vitamin C restores structural alterations of bones in heparin-induced osteoporosis. *Clin Rheumatol* 2003; 22(6):432–36.

SULFUR

Barrager E et al. A multicentered open-label trial on the safety and efficacy of methylsulfonylmethane in the treatment of seasonal allergic rhinitis. *J Altern Complement Med* 2002 Apr; 8(2):167–73.

Kim LS et al. Efficacy of methylsulfonylmethane (MSM) in osteoarthritis pain of the knee: a pilot clinical trial. *Osteoarthritis Cartilage* 2006 Mar; 14(3):286–94.

Mindell, Earl and Virginia Hopkins. *Dr. Earl Mindell's The Power of MSM*. McGraw-Hill, 2002.

ZINC

Birmingham CL, Gritzner S. How does zinc supplementation benefit anorexia nervosa? *Eat Weight Disord* 2006 Dec; 11(4):e109–11.

Overbeck S et al. Modulating the immune response by oral zinc supplementation: a single approach for multiple diseases. *Arch Immunol Ther Exp (Warsz)* 2008 Feb 5.

Herbal Remedies

ALOE VERA

Coats, Bill C. *Aloe Vera the New Millennium*. iUniverse, 2003.

Davis RH et al. Wound healing. Oral and topical activity of aloe vera. *J Am Pod Med Assoc* 1989; 79:559–62.

Grindlay D, Reynolds T. The aloe vera phenomenon: a review of the properties and modern uses of the leaf parenchyma gel. *J Ethnopharmacol* 1986; 16(2–3):117–51.

ARNICA

Jeffrey SL, Belcher HJ. Use of arnica to relieve pain after carpal-tunnel release surgery. *Altern Ther Health Med* 2002 Mar-Apr; 8(2):66–68.

Speight, Phyllis. *Arnica: The Remedy That Should Be in Every Home.* Random House, 2004.

ASTRAGALUS

Cho WC, Leung KN. In vitro and in vivo immunomodulating and immunorestorative effects of Astragalus membranaceus. J Ethnopharmacol 2007 Aug 15;113(1):132–41.

Kurashige A et al. Effects of astragali radix extract on carcinogenesis, cytokine production, and cytotoxicity in mice treated with a carcinogen, N-butyl-no-butanolnitrosoamine. *Cancer Invest* 1999; 17(1): 30–35.

Ma J et al. Mechanisms of the therapeutic effect of astragalus membranaceus on sodium and water retention in experimental heart failure. *Chin Med J* (Engl). 1998 Jan; 111(1):17–23.

Mao XQ et al. Astragalus polysaccharide reduces hepatic endoplasmic reticulum stress and restores glucose homeostasis in a diabetic KKAy mouse model. *Acta Pharmacol Sin* 2007 Dec; 28(12):1947–56.

BLACK COHOSH

Kligler B. Black cohosh. *Am Fam Physician* 2003; 68:114–16.

Oktem M et al. Black cohosh and fluoxetine in the treatment of postmenopausal symptoms: a prospective, randomized trial. *Adv Ther* 2007 Mar-Apr; 24(2): 448–61.

Pockaj BA et al. Pilot evaluation of black cohosh for the treatment of hot flashes in women. *Cancer Invest* 2004; 22(4):515–21.

Ruhlen RL et al. Black cohosh does not exert an estrogenic effect on the breast. *Nutr Cancer* 2007; 59(2): 269–77.

Walji R et al. Black cohosh (*Cimicifuga racemosa* [L.]Nutt): safety and efficacy for cancer patients. *Support Care Cancer* 2007 Aug; 15(8):913–21.

BOSWELLIA
Etzel R. Special extract of *Boswellia serrata* (H15) in the treatment of rheumatoid arthritis. *Phytomed* 1996; 3:91–94.

Gupta I et al. Effects of *Boswellia serrata* gum resin in patients with bronchial asthma: results of a double-blind, placebo-controlled, 6-week clinical study. *Eur J Med Res* 1998 Nov 17; 3(11):511–14.

BROMELAIN
Bromelain. *Alt Med Rev* 1998 Aug; 3:302–5.

Melis GB. Clinical experience with methoxybutropate vs. bromelin in the treatment of female pelvic inflammation. *Minerva Ginecol* 1990 Jul-Aug; 42(7–8):309–12.

Onken JE et al. Bromelain treatment decreases secretion of pro-inflammatory cytokines and chemokiens by colon biopsies in vitro. *Clin Immunol* 2008 Mar; 126(3):345–52.

BUTTERBUR
Diener HC et al. The first placebo-controlled trial of a special butterbur root extract for the prevention of migraine: reanalysis of efficacy criteria. *Eur Neurol* 2004; 51(2):89–97.

Elkins, Rita. *Natural Treatments for Urinary Incontinence: Using Butterbur and Other Natural Supplements to Treat Bladder Control Problems.* Woodland Health, 2000.

Lipton RB et al. *Petasite hybridus* root (butterbur) is an effective preventive treatment for migraine. *Neurology* 2004 Dec 28; 63912):2240–44.

CALENDULA

Basch E et al. Marigold (*Calendula officinalis*): an evidence-based systematic review by the Natural Standard Research Collaboration. *J Herb Pharmacother* 2006; 6(3–4):135–59.

Duran V et al. Results of the clinical examination of an ointment with marigold (*Calendula officinalis*) extract in the treatment of venous leg ulcers. *Int J Tissue React* 2005; 27(3):101–6.

CAPSAICIN

Deal CL et al. Treatment of arthritis with topical capsaicin: a double-blind trial. *Clin Ther* 1991; 13:383–95.

McCarthy GM, McCarthy DJ. Effect of topical capsaicin in the therapy of painful osteoarthritis of the hands. *J Rheumatol* 1992 Apr; 19(4):604–7.

CHAMOMILE

Cauffield JS, Forbes HJ. Dietary supplements used in the treatment of depression, anxiety, and sleep disorders. *Lippincotts Prim Care Pract* 1999 May-Jun; 3(3):290–304.

Srivastava JK, Gupta S. Antiproliferative and apoptotic effects of chamomile extract in various human cancer cells. *J Agric Food Chem* 2007 Nov 14; 55(23):9470–78.

CHASTE TREE BERRY

Roemheld-Hamm B. Chasteberry. *Am Fam Physician* 2005 Sep 1; 72(5):821–24.

Westphal LM et al. Double-blind, placebo-controlled study of Fertilityblend: a nutritional supplement for improving fertility in women. *Clin Exp Obstet Gynecol.* 2006; 33(4):205–8.

CINNAMON

Khan A et al. Cinnamon improves glucose and lipids of people with type 2 diabetes. *Diabetes Care* 2003 Dec; 26(12):3215–18.

Solomon TP, Blannin AK. Effects of short-term cinnamon ingestion on in vivo glucose tolerance. *Diabetes Obes Metab* 2007 Nov; 9(6):895–901.

CURCUMIN

Pari L, Murugan P. Effect of tetrahydrocurcumin on blood glucose, plasma insulin and hepatic key enzymes in streptozotocin induced diabetic rats. *J Basic Clin Physiol Pharmacol* 2005; 16(4):257–74.

Ringman JM et al. A potential role of the curry spice curcumin in Alzheimer's disease. *Curr Alzheimer Res* 2005 Apr; 2(2):131–36.

Singh S, Khar A. Biological effects of curcumin and its role in cancer chemoprevention and therapy. *Anticancer Agents Med Chem* 2006 May; 6(3):259–70.

DANDELION

Blumenthal M et al, eds. Dandelion root with herb. In *Herbal Medicine: Expanded Commission E Monographs.* Lippincott Williams & Wilkins, 2000.

Schutz K et al. Taraxacum—a review on its phytochemical and pharmacological profile. *J Ethnopharmacol* 2006 Oct 11; 107(3):313–23.

FEVERFEW

Diener HC et al. Efficacy and safety of 6.25 mg tid feverfew CO_2-extract (MIG-99) in migraine prevention— a randomized, double-blind, multicentre, placebo-controlled study. *Cephalalgia* 2005 Nov; 25(11):1031–41.

Eichenfield LF et al. Natural advances in eczema care. *Cutis* 2007 Dec; 80(6 Suppl):2–16.

FLAXSEED

Brooks JD et al. Supplementation with flaxseed alters estrogen metabolism in postmenopausal women to a greater extent than does supplementation with an equal amount of soy. *Am J Clin Nutr* 2004 Feb; 79(2):318–25.

Chen J et al. Flaxseed alone or in combination with tamoxifen inhibits MCF-7 breast tumor growth in ovariectomized athymic mice with high circulating levels of estrogen. *Exp Biol Med* 2007 Sep; 232(8):1071–80.

Patade A et al. Flaxseed reduces total and LDL cholesterol concentrations in Native American postmenopausal women. *J Womens Health (Larchmt)* 2008 Mar 8.

GARLIC

Fani MM et al. Inhibitory activity of garlic (*Allium sativum*) extract on multidrug-resistant *Streptococcus mutans*. *J Indian Soc Pedod Prev Dent* 2007 Oct-Dec; 25(4):164–8.

Hronek M et al. Antifungal effect in selected natural compounds and probiotics and their possible use in prophylaxis of vulvovaginitis. *Ceska Gynekol* 2005 Sep; 70(5):395–99.

Mennella JA et al. Garlic ingestion by pregnant women alters the odor of amniotic fluid. *Chem Senses* 1995; 20:207–9.

Weber ND et al. In vitro virucidal effects of *Allium sativum* (garlic) extract and compounds. *Planta Med* 1992 Oct; 58(5):417–23.

GINGER
Bryer E. A literature review of the effectiveness of ginger in alleviating mild-to-moderate nausea and vomiting of pregnancy. *J Midwifery Womens Health* 2005; 50(1):e1–e3.

Mahesh R et al. Cancer chemotherapy-induced nausea and vomiting: role of mediators, development of drugs and treatment methods. *Pharmazie* 2005; 60(2):83–96.

Schulick, Paul. *Ginger: Common Spice and Wonder Drug*. Hohm Press, 2001.

GINKGO
Hilton M, Stuart E. Ginkgo biloba for tinnitus. *Cochrane Database Syst Rev* 2004; (2):CD003852.

Solomon PR et al. Ginkgo for memory enhancement: a randomized controlled trial. *JAMA* 2002 Aug 21; 288(7):835–40.

Wu Y et al. Ginkgo biloba extract improves coronary blood flow in healthy elderly adults: role of endothelium-dependent vasodilation. *Phytomedicine* 2008 Mar; 15(3):164–69.

GINSENG
Taylor, David. *Ginseng, the Divine Root*. Algonquin Books, 2006.

Vuksan V et al. Korean red ginseng (*Panax ginseng*) improves glucose and insulin regulation in well-controlled, type 2 diabetes: results of a randomized, double-blind, placebo-controlled study of efficacy and safety. *Nutr Metab Cardiovasc Dis* 2008 Jan; 18(1): 46–56.

GREEN TEA

Brown MD. Green tea (*Camellia sinensis*) extract and its possible role in the prevention of cancer. *Alt Med Rev* 1999; 4(5):360–70.

Mitscher, Lester and Victoria Toews. *The Green Tea Book*. Avery, 2007.

Setiawan VW et al. Protective effect of green tea on the risks of chronic gastritis and stomach cancer. *Int J Cancer* 2001; 92(4):600–604.

Suzuki Y et al. Green tea and the risk of breast cancer: pooled analysis of two prospective studies in Japan. *Br J Cancer* Apr 5, 2004; 90(7):1361–63.

HAWTHORN

Pittler M et al. Hawthorn extract for treating chronic heart failure. *Cochrane Database Syst Rev*. 2008 Jan 23; (1):CD005312.

HORSE CHESNUT

Diehm C et al. Comparison of leg compression stocking and oral horse-chestnut seed extract therapy in patients with chronic venous insufficiency. *Lancet* 1996; 347:292–94.

Pittler MH et al. Horse-chestnut seed extract for chronic venous insufficiency. A criteria-based systemic review. *Arch Dermatol* 1998; 134:1356–60.

PEPPERMINT

McKay DL, Blumberg JB. A review of the bioactivity and potential health benefits of peppermint tea (*Mentha piperita* L.). *Phytother Res* 2006 Aug; 20(8):619–33.

Westfall RE. Use of anti-emetic herbs in pregnancy: women's choices, and the question of safety and efficacy. *Complement Ther Nurs Midwifery* 2004 Feb;10(1):30–6.

PSYLLIUM

Bijkerk CJ et al. Systematic review: the role of different types of fibre in the treatment of irritable bowel syndrome. *Aliment Pharmacol Ther* 2004 Feb 1; 19(3):245–51.

Coon JT et al. *Trifolium pratense* isoflavones in the treatment of menopausal hot flushes: a systematic review and meta-analysis. *Phytomedicine* 2007 Feb; 14(2–3): 153–59.

Geller SE, Studee L. Soy and red clover for mid-life and aging. *Climacteric* 2006 Aug; 9(4):245–63.

Hidalgo LA et al. The effect of red clover isoflavones on menopausal symptoms, lipids and vaginal cytology in menopausal women: a randomized, double-blind, placebo-controlled study. *Gynecol Endocrinol* 2005 Nov; 21(5):257–64.

Occhiuto F et al. Effects of phytoestrogenic isoflavones from red clover (*Trifolium pratense* L.) on experimental osteoporosis. *Phytother Red* 2007 Feb; 21(2):130–34.

ST. JOHN'S WORT

Brenner R et al. Comparison of an extract of hypericum (LI 160) and sertraline in the treatment of depression: a double-blind, randomized pilot study. *Clin Ther* 2000: 22(4):411–19.

McIntosh, Kenneth. *"Natural" Alternatives to Antidepressants: St. John's Wort, Kava Kava, and Others.* Mason Crest, 2007.

Stevinson C, Ernst E. A pilot study of *Hypericum perforatum* for the treatment of premenstrual syndrome. *Br J Obstet Gynaecol* 2000; 107:870–76.

TEA TREE OIL
Lawless, Julia. *Tea Tree Oil: Nature's Miracle Healer.* Thorsons, 2001.

Park H et al. Antibacterial effect of tea-tree oil on methicillin-resistant Staphylococcus aureus biofilm formation of the tympanostomy tube: an in vitro study. *In Vivo* 2007 Nov-Dec; 21(6):1027–30.

UVA URSI
Jahodar L et al. Antimicrobial effect of arbutin and an extract of the leaves of *Arctostaphylos uva-ursi* in vitro. *Cesk Farm* 1985 Jun; 34(5):174–78.

Matsuda H et al. Pharmacological studies on leaf of *Arctostaphylos uva-ursi* (L) Spreng. *J Pharm Soc Japan* 1992; 112:673–77.

VALERIAN
American Academy of Sleep Medicine. Many insomniacs turn to valerian and melatonin to help them sleep. *Science Daily.* Retrieved March 10, 2008, from http://www.sciencedaily.com /releases/2007/ 07/070703171930.htm.

Hadley S, Petry JJ. Valerian. *Am Fam Phys* 2003 Apr; 67:1755–58.

Ziegler G et al. Efficacy and tolerability of valerian extract LI 156, compared with oxazepam in the treatment of nonorganic insomnia: a randomized, double-blind, comparative clinical study. *Eur J Med Res* 2002; 25:480–86.

Amino Acids and Miscellaneous Supplements

AMINO ACIDS

Griffith RS et al. Success of L-lysine therapy in frequently recurrent herpes simplex infection. Treatment and prophylaxis. *Dermatologica* 1987; 175(4):183–90.

Gupta RC et al. Taurine analogues; a new class of thera-peutics: retrospect and prospects. *Curr Med Chem* 2005; 12(17):2021–39.

Kendler BS. Supplemental conditionally essential nutrients in cardiovascular disease therapy. *J Cardiovasc Nurs* 2006 Jan-Feb; 21(1):9–16.

Mason R. 200 mg of Zen: L-theanine boosts alpha waves, promotes alert relaxation. *Alt Complem Ther* 2001 Apr; 7:91–95.

Rossini M et al. Double-blind, multicenter trial comparing acetyl L-carnitine with placebo in the treatment of fibromyalgia patients. *Clin Exp Rheumatol* 2007 Mar-Apr; 25(2):182–88.

CAROTENOIDS

Delgado-Vargas F et al. Natural pigments: carotenoids, anthocyanins, and betalains—characteristics, biosyn-thesis, processing, and stability. *Crit Rev Food Sci Nutr* 2000 May; 40(3):173–289.

Krinsky NI. Carotenoids as antioxidants. *Nutrition* 2001 Oct; 17(10):815–17.

COENZYME Q_{10}

Baggio E et al. Italian multicenter study on the safety and

efficacy of coenzyme Q_{10} as adjunctive therapy in heart failure. CoQ_{10} Drug Surveillance Investigators. *Mol Aspects Med* 1994; 15(Suppl):s287–94.

Khatta M et al. The effect of coenzyme Q_{10} in patients with congestive heart failure. *Ann Int Med* 2000; 132(8): 636–40.

Premkumar VG et al. Effect of coenzyme Q_{10}, riboflavin and niacin on serum CEA and CA 15–3 levels in breast cancer patients undergoing tamoxifen therapy. *Biol Pharm Bull* 2007 Feb; 30(2):387–70.

Wexler, Barbara. *Coenzyme Q_{10}: The Essence of Energy.* Woodland Publishing, 2007.

DHEA

Allolio B et al. DHEA: why, when, and how much—DHEA replacement in adrenal insufficiency. *Ann Endocrinol (Paris)* 2007 Sep; 68(4):268–73.

Gurnell EM et al. Long-term DHEA replacement in primary adrenal insufficiency: a randomized, controlled trial. *J Clin Endocrinol Metab* 2008 Feb; 93(2):400–409.

Moore, Neecie. *The Facts About DHEA.* Alethia Corp, 2005.

5-HTP

Cangiano C et al. Eating behavior and adherence to dietary prescriptions in obese adult subjects treated with 5-hydroxytryptophan. *Am J Clin Nutr* 1992 Nov; 56(5):863–67.

Murray, Michael, ND. *5-HTTP: The Natural Way to Overcome Depression, Obesity, and Insomnia.* Bantam, 1999.

GLUCOSAMINE

McAlindon TE et al. Glucosamine and chondroitin for treatment of osteoarthritis: a systematic quality assessment and meta-analysis. *JAMA* 2000; 283:1469–75.

Toews, Victoria Dolby. *User's Guide to Glucosamine and Chondroitin: Don't Be a Dummy: Become an Expert on What Glucosamine and Chondroitin Can Do.* Basic Health Publications, 2002.

MELATONIN

Lemoine P et al. Prolonged-release melatonin improves sleep quality and morning alertness in insomnia patients aged 55 years and older and has no withdrawal effects. *J Sleep Res* 2007 Dec; 16(4):372–80.

Melatonin—A Medical Dictionary, Bibliography, and Annotated Research Guide to Internet References. ICON Health Publications, 2004.

Pandi-Peruimal TK et al. Role of the melatonin system in the control of sleep: therapeutic implications. *CNS Drugs* 2007; 21(12):995–1018.

MSM

Jacob, Stanley W., MD and Jeremy Appleton. *MSM: The Definitive Guide: The Nutritional Breakthrough for Arthritis, Allergies, and More.* Freedom Press, 2002.

Kim LS et al. Efficacy of methylsulfonylmethane (MSM) in osteoarthritis pain of the knee: a pilot clinical trial. *Osteoarthritis Cartilage* 2006 Mar; 14(3): 286–94.

SAM-e

Adenosylmethionine (SAMe) for osteoarthritis. *J Fam Pract* 2002; 51(5):425–30.

Jacobsen S et al. Oral S-adenosylmethionine in primary fibromyalgia: double-blind clinical evaluation. *Scand J Rheumatol* 1991; 20:294–302.

Mitchell, Deborah. *The Sam-e Solution: The Essential Guide to the Revolutionary Antidepressant Supplement.* Grand Central Publishing, 1999.